Social Theory, Health and Healthcare

Social Theory, Health and Healthcare

Orla McDonnell
Maria Lohan
Abbey Hyde
Sam Porter

palgrave
macmillan

First published 2009 by
PALGRAVE MACMILLAN

Palgrave Macmillan in the UK is an imprint of Macmillan Publishers Limited,
registered in England, company number 785998, of Houndmills, Basingstoke,
Hampshire RG21 6XS.

Palgrave Macmillan in the US is a division of St Martin's Press LLC,
175 Fifth Avenue, New York, NY 10010.

Palgrave Macmillan is the global academic imprint of the above companies
and has companies and representatives throughout the world.

Palgrave® and Macmillan® are registered trademarks in the United States,
the United Kingdom, Europe and other countries.

ISBN 978-1-4039-8953-6   ISBN 978-1-137-06215-4 (eBook)
DOI 10.1007/978-1-137-06215-4

This book is printed on paper suitable for recycling and made from fully
managed and sustained forest sources. Logging, pulping and manufacturing
processes are expected to conform to the environmental regulations of the
country of origin.

A catalogue record for this book is available from the British Library.

A catalog record for this book is available from the Library of Congress.

10   9   8   7   6   5   4   3   2   1
18   17 16 15 14 13 12 11 10 09

Maria Lohan would like to dedicate this publication to her late parents John and Maureen Lohan.

Abbey Hyde would like to dedicate this publication to the late Billy Murphy (1899–1979), Knockmullane, Innishannon, Co. Cork.

Sam Porter: Do Siobhán agus Ewan: bualtraí uair amháin eile.

Contents

Social Theory, Health and Healthcare

We are living in times when health and healthcare are becoming ever more controversial and contested. While once it was the case that when a person got sick it was seen as the luck of the draw, now we try to find out what it was in their circumstances and lifestyle that led to their sickness. When once we just did what the doctor told us, now we seek out information on the internet and use that to question medical decisions. When once we thought of health visitors as innocent and kindly, now we wonder whether they are spying on us to see if we are good enough parents. When once we took it for granted that vaccinations would be good for our children, now we wonder if they might be worse than the diseases they are preventing. In short, when once things were simple, they are now far more complicated. Or, maybe it just seems that way – whatever the case, we are certainly more aware of the complexities and controversies surrounding health and healthcare.

What is going on? Well, that is the question that this book seeks to answer. It starts from the premise that the only way to do this is to broaden our view beyond technical explanations about disease aetiology, medical knowledge, health visiting practices, or the biochemistry of vaccines, and to focus on the social context in which these things are occurring. One way of doing this is to examine each controversy in its own terms in order to find out about the experiences, interpretations, relationships and actions of the people involved. The problem with that is that we would have to reinvent the explanatory wheel for every case that we look at. It is, therefore, far more sensible to identify general principles that can be applied (albeit in modified forms to suit the question at hand) to explain relationships, actions and experiences in all sorts of different cases. Those general principles are what we call social theory.

The objective of this book is to introduce the reader to the principles of the main schools of social theory and to demonstrate how they may be applied to offer deeper understandings of health and healthcare. The study of health and healthcare is a wide ranging subject which is spread across many disciplines. Social theory can help make sense of all this – the identification of general principles allows us to see the links in the seemingly diverse areas of healthcare. Social theory is also a broad enterprise, which is sometimes viewed as divorced from the descriptive work involved in research. In this book we wish to show how the theoretical and empirical dimensions of research are interlinked. Theories are important in terms of how researchers conceive of their research field and in terms of what they look for. Theories help us to move beyond description to offer explanations. This is not to say they provide eternal truths – as the social world changes, theories are revised or pushed in different directions or, indeed, revamped. To reflect this, we have chosen to organize this book based on a selection of the main schools of social theory. The theoretical perspectives covered include structural functionalism as applied to 'social capital' and the 'sick role'; political economy as applied to inequalities in health and the 'proletarianization' of medicine; social interactionism as applied to the 'social construction' of health and illness as well as healthcare work; poststructuralism as applied to 'governance of the self' as well as healthcare and surveillance; critical realism as applied to a critique of genetics, the disability debate and inequalities in health, as well as a critique of using the randomized control trial (RCT) as the 'gold standard' in the evaluation of healthcare; feminist theory as applied to the gendered patterning of both health and healthcare work; and finally the sociology of science and technology as applied to the role of genetic technologies in the field of medicine.

In each chapter, we outline the basic principles of the theory to hand, as well as some of the main points of contention about it. We then show how these social theories are applied in empirical research specific to health and healthcare issues. Of course, given our ambition of demonstrating how social theory can be applied to understandings of health and healthcare, the book could have been written from the other way around – by specifying particular health or healthcare issues and working our way back to theory. However, we hope that by beginning with the theories and showing how they can be applied, we are able to make what might seem difficult and abstract ideas understandable, allowing the reader to evaluate them in terms of their usefulness in offering explanations and in raising questions that have political, practical and moral import for our understandings of health and healthcare.

Because different social theories show phenomena in different ways, more than one branch of social theory may be needed to create a rounded or more critical picture of any given question relating to health. On the other hand, it is sometimes the case that there is very little compatibility between different theoretical approaches to the same phenomenon, and it becomes a matter of choosing between them. In dealing with a limited number of theoretical positions in depth in this book, we hope we have provided the reader with sufficient information to make such choices if needs be. Through a quick glance at the index, the reader will find that some of the major contemporary concerns of social scientists' research on health and healthcare come up under the different theories. While we provide pointers in each of the chapters to these cross-cutting themes, we felt it would be helpful to use this introduction to tease out some of them.

Let us begin with the *doctor–patient relationship*. In Chapter 1, the functionalist theory of the 'sick role' as developed through Talcott Parsons' empirical observations of doctor–patient relationships in the USA in the 1950s suggests a consensus around the principle of 'doctor knows best'. Parsons' characterization of the relationship between doctor and patient as consensual mirrors his general theory of society, which is based on the idea of a harmonious fit between the functional needs of society and its institutional structures. For Parsons, the nature of the doctor–patient relationship functions to fit the wider needs of society in the sense that professional dominance and patient acquiescence allows sickness (and the return from sickness to normal 'productive' social roles) to be managed in a manner that does not interfere with normal social activities, most particularly work-related activities, which are held by both sides as a collective good. However, this chapter also charts how changing healthcare philosophies and policies have recast the doctor–patient relationship from a Parsonian consensual model to a model that recognizes the important role of negotiation between the players involved (Mead and Bower 2000).

The poststructuralist theories associated with the French philosopher Michel Foucault also help explain an acceptance of, and trust in, contemporary medical authority through a historical analysis of the development of a new expert system (medicine) and expert workers (doctors). It is argued that these expert systems flourished in new forms of government from the eighteenth century, which involved the development of scientific knowledge about the health of individuals and populations, and the use of that knowledge to regulate them. Unlike the functionalist perspective, poststructuralist theory is more critical of the pervasive regulatory powers of modern medicine. In terms of new directions, we show how Foucault's ideas are taken up and developed in research to show how the contemporary ideal of the 'healthy self' is more problematic and politically relevant than health promotional discourse would lead us to believe.

Political economists are also critical of medical dominance, but through an explicitly economic understanding of society that concentrates on class conflict. Political economy links an analysis of the organization of healthcare to the broader organization of the economy. In particular, it shows how changes in the ownership and organization of healthcare systems involving the introduction of market values into healthcare are turning health into a commodity. The consequences of this are manifold and felt right across the organization of healthcare. Specifically, it is argued in relation to doctor–patient relationships, that the ethos of professionalism (expert driven, universal and impartial care) which functionalists assumed to be a central to the medical profession, is being eroded by the introduction of market driven principles into healthcare: Physician autonomy to choose a treatment path for a patient is strongly determined by economic decision-making made at an institutional level (whether or not to invest in particular forms of care pathways) and/or the patient's ability to pay for healthcare. The political economy perspective also offers a more critical focus on the rise of 'patient-centred' care because it is argued that it has been subsumed by market-oriented policies, which construct patients as 'consumers' who have to purchase good healthcare. In turn, this encourages privatization and competition in the healthcare market, thus absolving the state of its responsibility to provide universal healthcare, reversing the general consensus of many post-war industrialized/industrializing societies about the state's central role in caring for the health of its citizens. This theme is also explored in Chapter 4 on poststructuralist thinking, but in a way that focuses less on the state and more on the diverse and, sometimes, contradictory ways that power works in enrolling our support for such practices.

A number of the chapters highlight the potential for some theories to increase our understanding of *patient experiences*. In Chapter 6, we show how feminist writers link the historical oppression of women to the construction of women's bodies and minds in medical discourses as pathological or potentially pathological. Feminist work has critiqued the power of medicine and the medical profession over women's bodies and this has given rise to a large body of work that seeks to explore women's experiences of healthcare and includes phenomenological research (inspired also by Social Interaction Theory as outlined in Chapter 3). We suggest that future research is also likely to continue addressing the tension between focusing on women's *embodied experiences* on the one hand, and the interpretation of women's experiences as products of cultural discourses and institutional practices on the other. Some feminist thinkers (e.g., Kruks 2001, Davis 2007) argue that the way forward is to begin from the experiences of women, but to theorize these in relation to cultural discourses and institutional arrangements and the socio-political contexts in which they arise. Chapters 3 and 6 thus highlight patients' voices on health and healthcare, while Chapter 4 on poststructuralism raises questions about the limits to patient-centred models of communication, patient empowerment and the role of experiential knowledge as a legitimate source of authority in therapeutic decision-making and policy decisions about the governance of healthcare.

Chapter 2 (Political Economy) and Chapter 6 (Feminist Theory) throw up interesting theories on *professionals' experience of working in healthcare*. Chapter 2 evaluates the evidence for and against the theory of the 'proletarianization' of the medical workforce, which challenges the notion that physicians are dominant in the healthcare workforce, controlling both their own work and that of other healthcare. It is argued that across advanced Western capitalist societies, cost-saving strategies, new management principles and the professionalization of other healthcare workers have eroded the power and autonomy of medicine. Whilst one writer's somewhat provocative analysis of contemporary medical work as being akin to assembly line factory work – 'working on the factory floor with an MD degree' (Stoeckle 1987: 250) does not accord with most analyses, the proletarianization thesis does allow us to ask questions about the impact of modernization on healthcare provision and also opens doors for analyzing doctors' (and other healthcare workers') own perceptions of their changing roles and identities in contemporary healthcare.

Feminist theory has also long claimed to provide a solid analytical framework through which to view professional and, particularly, interprofessional *nurse–doctor relationships* in healthcare. In the words of Wicks (1998: 4), feminist theory has 'shone like a beacon onto the nurse/doctor relationship and illuminated the unequal and often exploitative power relations…It raised vital questions such as who gives the orders and who takes them, who does the stimulating work and who does the drudge work, and who gets paid more and who gets paid less.' However, the changing gender demographics of medicine, in particular, muddies the picture somewhat. For example, Porter's (1992) analysis of relations between nurses and doctors indicates that while gender continues to be an issue in the relationship between the two parties, its effects are moderated by an increasing proportion of women in medicine.

Moving along to the important theme of *health inequalities*, the fact that social factors remain the most powerful predictor of one's expected age of death (or lifespan) is perhaps the most compelling argument for the need for social theory in health and healthcare research. The persistence of health inequalities between the most well off and least well off in many societies remains the major health and healthcare dilemma of our time. Chapter 2 shows that the last few decades of social science and epidemiological research indicate the particular salience of political economy theories to understanding this problem. This perspective emphasizes the role of material factors such as low income, unemployment, poor housing, poor communities and exposure to hazards in explaining the poorer health of individuals in the lower social classes relative to those in the higher social classes. In addition, Chapters 1 and 2 highlight the ways in which traditional Marxist theory has been drawn into productive debates with neo-fucntionalist theories of social capital concerning psychosocial explanations of inequalities in health. Chapter 2 points to innovative approaches that seek to combine both material and psychosocial perspectives over the life-course in order to understand the complex pathways that link social inequality to health inequality in people's lives. Nonetheless, critical realists (Chapter 5) observe the need for deeper causative explanations than those currently being offered. They argue that although observations that poverty and inequality are associated with inequalities in health are significant findings, they are not sufficient, in that they cannot explain why social inequalities are so stark, and getting starker. Instead, they argue that there is a need to return to Marxist theory in order to uncover the underlying causative mechanisms that generate these inequalities. Critical realists, therefore, are concerned with understanding the processes that can lead to political and economic transformations in societies to address the underlying causes of inequalities in those societies.

The term 'medicalization' was first introduced by Irving Zola (1972) who applied it to a number of issues, namely: the expansion of areas deemed to be relevant to medicine; the retention by medicine of absolute control over specific technical procedures; the retention by medicine of access to taboo areas; and the expansion of what in medicine is considered to be relevant to the good practice of life. The concept of *medicalization*, therefore, intersects with a number of the classical theories introduced in this book. Medicine plays a formative role in what Foucault understands as uniquely modern forms of power (Chapter 4, poststructuralism). In *The Birth of the Clinic*, Foucault ([1973] 1976) charts a critical historical framework for the growth of medical authority in people's lives. Under the auspices of public health in the later eighteenth century, the 'medical gaze' penetrated the social space and instilled a generalized medical consciousness about the role of health and good living. Later on in the nineteenth century, the 'clinical gaze' was institutionalized in the birth of the hospital clinic where patients could be observed and examined, cases recorded and compared, treatments administered and monitored. The concept of medicalization is further developed in feminist theory and research (Chapter 6). In particular, feminist research is critical of the way in which everyday aspects of life such as pregnancy, birth, menopause and ageing have come under the jurisdiction of medicine. Moving to Chapter 5, we show how the concept of medicalization as developed in Conrad's (1999) critique of an over-reliance on genetics in explaining complicated multi-causal illnesses may be linked to the classical critical theory critique of 'specific aetiology' – that every disease has a specific cause. Conrad similarly critiques a monogenic model of disease causation, whereby a gene or genetic mutation is regarded as determining a disease or behaviour (see also the discussion of 'geneticization' (Lippman 1998) in Chapter 7). Finally, in Chapter 7, the contemporary processes of medicalization are captured by the concept of 'biomedicalization' (Clarke *et al.* 2003) to describe the emerging bio-industrial complex supporting the commercialization of genetic research.

Chapter 7 introduces an innovative group of broadly constructivist social theories of science and technology known as Science and Technology Studies (STS), which are increasingly been applied to understanding the role of *technology within health and healthcare*. Clearly, technologies impact on our understanding of health and our embodied identities, from simple adjustments such as the wearing of spectacles to more permanent changes such as sex changes, organ transplantation, and medical and surgical treatments targeted to 'risk groups' to pre-empt the development of disease, most notably in relation to breast and prostate cancer. Clearly, also, scientific and technological innovations associated with molecular biology and genetics, biotechnologies, transplant medicine and magnetic resonance imaging impact on the delivery of healthcare. However, as critical realists have pointed out (Chapter 5), there is much more that contributes to the success or failure of technologies in healthcare settings than the characteristics of the technology itself. An important feature of social theories that fall under STS is that they challenge prevalent views of technology as *external* to social relations but which nonetheless have a *determining* influence in our social relations (known as technological determinism). Thus, SST expands the role of social scientists and ethicists from merely analyzing the social *consequences* of technology on health and healthcare, to entering 'the belly of the beast' and analyzing the social organization of the production and implementation of technology. A social shaping perspective on technology, in particular, rejects a linear deterministic view of technology and instead develops an interest in the construction and organization of the science and technology, emphasizing how social and economic interests influence how science and technology is developed and how, in turn, they impact on society. This draws our attention to the wider political and social contexts that shape technologies.

More recent social theories of science and technology, most notably the Social Construction of Technology (SCOT) and Actor Network Theory (ANT), are concerned to develop a more symbiotic understanding of the mutual shaping of society and technology. Both SCOT and ANT approaches conceive of technologies using the metaphor of a 'network'. Technologies are made up of social and technical elements, which ANT refers to as 'actors'. For example, scientists and researchers, the tools and materials that they use, commercial and public funders and their resources, as well as users and potential users, are all seen as actors in the network. While there are clear theoretical distinctions between these approaches, which we draw out in the text, both share a methodological principle that we cannot determine prior to empirical research what will determine the way a technology is shaped, how it will become part of our everyday lives or routine institutional practices, or how its effects will be distributed in society. In the application of these theories to understanding health and healthcare, we focus particularly on genetic technologies, which offer us interesting insights into the way that these novel, and sometimes controversial, technologies shape our understandings of health and our expectations about the future of healthcare.

Finally, two of the chapters (Chapters 3 and 5) directly address the *methodological implications* of social theories for researching health and healthcare. Chapter 3 describes social interaction theory as a broad theoretical perspective that emphasizes the significance and centrality of subjective meanings associated with social actions and institutions. This theory promotes an interpretive understanding of society as socially produced through the small-scale interactions that occur between individuals in everyday life. Since social action theorists, or interpretivists, broadly view humans as active in shaping their world, this has implications for how they view social change. Individuals are considered to be knowledgable actors and, as such, change is possible from the bottom-up rather than being imposed from above. In a crude sense, interpretivists are less concerned with explaining social processes through the influence of large-scale institutions on people's lives, but rather are concerned with people's subjective meanings and with individual agency. Critical realists (Chapter 5), by contrast, argue for a methodological approach that can combine an analysis of subjective understandings and social structures. Therefore, this methodological approach calls for research designs that allow for a circular process of analysis between individuals' interpretations and actions which affect social structures and the underlying structural aspects of society that, in turn, influence those interpretations and actions. This leads critical realists to be sceptical of explanations that view human behaviour as determined by a single factor. An example of this reductionism that is dealt with in this chapter concerns those explanations that see our behaviour and our health as being determined by our genes.

Inevitably, there are additional social theories that we have not had space to develop in this book. For example, whilst risk is present as a theme in the book (especially in Chapter 4), theories of risk are not developed in-depth and readers may wish to refer to the journal, *Health, Risk and Society*. Also, whilst we have not given a whole chapter to critical theory, we have dealt with two theoretical approaches that overlap its concerns, namely political economy theory and critical realism. Theories of the body are also the subject of a substantial field of research that opens up new insights for the sociology of health. The sociology of the body draws on a diverse range of theoretical perspectives, including some of those discussed in this book, in particular, phenomenological theory (Chapter 3), poststructuralism (Chapter 4), critical realism (Chapter 5) and feminism (Chapter 6). How we conceive of the body other than as a biological entity is discussed in Chapter 6 on feminism and in Chapter 5 (critical realism) in relation to theorizing disability.

This brings us to another important sub-disciplinary field in social theory, which is Disability Studies. While social theories of disability are not dealt with in any great depth in this book, the 'social model' of disability (which developed not only in opposition to the biomedical model but also as a critique of some of the classical social theories discussed in this book, including Parsons' theory of the sick role discussed in Chapter 1, and Symbolic Interactionism outlined in Chapter 3) posits particular challenges for how we understand the intersection between the body and society as discussed in Chapter 5.

Before embarking on this book, the perceptive reader may be tempted to ask 'So what? Why should I invest my precious time and energy absorbing what does not look the most amenable body of knowledge, when I could practice or research just as well within health or healthcare without all this intellectual baggage?' Well, our answer is that your practice or research would be the poorer for a lack of social theory. We say this for at least two reasons. First, because our health is so deeply bound up with our position in society, and because healthcare is at its core a social activity, it is impossible to understand either fully unless we can understand the social dynamics associated with them. In other words, social knowledge as codified in general precepts, i.e., social theory, is a core part of the knowledge base for those who seek to gain an adequate understanding of health, illness and care. Second, whether we recognize it or not, we all make assumptions about the nature of the social world around us, and act on the basis of those assumptions. Acting on the basis of assumptions that we do not even recognize we are making is not the firmest grounding for either practice or research. In this book, we present a number of models in which those assumptions are made explicit. You may choose to accept some of them and not others; you may seek to combine the best of different models; or you may even reject them all (there are plenty more theories out there that we have not covered). What is important is that social theories are a resource to help you reflect on what you think is going on and why in the areas of health and healthcare in which you are interested. If all this book does is encourage readers of different scholarly backgrounds and health disciplines to examine their own presumptions about how the world is organized, then it will have served a useful task.

CHAPTER 1

Structural Functionalism, Health and Healthcare

Introduction

In this chapter, we begin with the work of the classical theorist and one of the key founding figures of sociology, Émile Durkheim (1858–1917). His work is essentially concerned with how societies reproduce themselves through collective belief systems and practices, and how individual members are collectively bound by values and norms that govern societal practices. In turn, these practices regulate society and create a sense of social solidarity. Like other classical theorists, he was interested in understanding the transition from traditional to modern society in order to explain the impact of social change. We go on to discuss structural functionalism as a distinct body of modern social theory, which represents one particular line of influence from the classical work of Durkheim. Within the sub-disciplinary field of the sociology of medicine, Talcott Parsons (1902–1979) is the most noted of the structuralist functionalist theorists. (Robert Merton is another central figure in the development of this theoretical perspective and his work is discussed in Chapter 7 in relation to the sociology of knowledge and science). A central thread that links the classical legacy of Durkheim to structural functionalism is the idea that shared norms and values are fundamental to society functioning as a cohesive whole. This core idea became the hallmark of Parsons' work and, more generally, has led to the characterization of structural functionalism as a 'consensus theory' of society. An example of what we mean by this is the emphasis that Parsons places on the function that social institutions such as medicine play in meeting the needs of society to maintain social and political stability.

While structural functionalism dominated American social theory in the 1950s and 1960s, more critical perspectives concerned

11

with unmasking the tensions and conflicts behind apparently stable and harmonious social and political structures became more mainstream by the mid-1970s. However, some sociologists have noted a revival in Durkheimian sociology since the 1990s in the expanding field of 'social capital' research (Blaxter 2000, Turner 2003). In the discussion on the application of structural functionalism to understanding health, we will explore the contribution of social capital theory to debates about the pervasive problem of health inequalities, a theme that is further developed under the perspective of 'political economy' theories in Chapter 2 and 'critical realism' in Chapter 5. We then turn to the classical account of the doctor–patient relationship offered by Parsons in his 'sick role' theory, which has perhaps more than any other theory earned sociology a place in healthcare research. However, while the sick role remains a remarkably stable concept in medical discourse it has become less popular as an analytical concept in sociological theory and, as we go on to discuss, new lines of enquiry and new explanatory frameworks have overtaken it.

Principles of structural functionalism

Let us start with a definition of the term 'structural functionalism'. Structuralism refers to a view of society which asserts that people's behaviour is structured according to a set of rules or laws. Functionalism is the view that society is a system made up of interconnected parts, each of which functions in a specific way to maintain the system as a whole (Porter 1998). These ideas were developed by the nineteenth-century French sociologist, Émile Durkheim. Durkheim's work is concerned with defining sociology as a distinct discipline that could emulate the so-called 'hard sciences'. He describes sociology as the study of 'social facts' relating to social structures – the work of sociology is to explain patterns that emerge in the social world ('social facts') by linking the *determining cause* of these social phenomena to their *social effect*. Social structures constrain individual actions and, therefore, human deeds cannot be explained solely in relation to individual motivations or behaviours. Moreover, since society is more than simply the sum of the self-interests of individuals, the problem of how society is socially integrated (what ties its members together), particularly as it undergoes processes of change, is a central concern in Durkheim's work.

The social division of labour

Like other classical social theorists, Durkheim is concerned with the way in which the modern processes of urbanization and industrialization break down traditional ways of living. In *The Division of Labour in Society* ([1893] 1964), Durkheim explains that traditional and modern societies are integrated differently. Traditional societies (e.g., agrarian subsistence societies where the family is the dominant economic unit) are structured by a simple 'division of labour', meaning that people perform similar functions to each other, which creates a shared bond within society based on common experiences and shared beliefs (Ritzer and Goodman 2003). He refers to this form of social integration as 'mechanical solidarity'. Modern society, on the other hand, is characterized by a more complex division of labour where people perform specialized tasks in an ever-widening range of structures and institutions. Here we need only to think about the growth in institutions associated with the welfare state in the twentieth century and the important role that these play in social protection, education and health, functions previously associated with the traditional institution of the family. Durkheim characterizes the social integration that arises from mutual dependency created by the more complex division of labour in modern society as 'organic solidarity'.

In modern society social bonds based on a shared way of life are inevitably weaker and social integration is a function of the mutual dependency of people's needs and 'the mutual relationships between [specialized] functions' (Durkheim in Calhoun *et al.* 2002: 145). For Durkheim, this interdependency is consolidated through the 'network of ties' that becomes institutionalized in society over time. As society undergoes rapid social and economic change, the norms, values and beliefs that guide people in the conduct of their everyday lives and that reproduce a sense of collective belonging are weakened. This gives rise to a state of 'anomie' – a concept that Durkheim uses to explain the breakdown in traditional social norms. In this situation, individuals are set adrift and isolated from the kind of common bonds that are formed in, for example, family and kin networks, community and in the work place. Durkheim suggests that the complex division of labour in modern society, which has the potential to create new forms of solidarity based on the interdependency of needs and specialized functions, also has 'pathological' tendencies in the sense of producing unhealthy societies evidenced, for example, by rising rates of suicide.

Conceptualizing suicide as a problem of social integration

Durkheim develops his argument on the problem of social integration in modern society in his study of suicide ([1897] 1951). In this study, which best illustrates his concept of anomie, Durkheim offers an important sociological insight that suicide, more commonly understood as an individual act of self-destruction, can be explained in relation to underlying social factors. In explaining the differential rates of suicides cross-culturally and over time, he argues that too little or too much social integration and social regulation creates the social conditions for different patterns of suicide (Ritzer and Goodman 2003). To this end, he identifies four types of suicide. The two dominant types of suicide in modern societies are 'egotistic' and 'anomic' suicide. Durkheim associates these patterns of suicide with low levels of social integration and regulation in societies marked by individualism and disruptive social change. In the case of the former pattern, suicide is the result of the weakening of social bonds, whereas the latter is associated with the kind of social disconnection that arises from radical social and economic change, which weakens the hold that traditional norms have in regulating individual behaviour. Durkheim identifies 'altruistic' and 'fatalistic' suicide as the dominant patterns in traditional societies, which are more highly integrated and regulated. In traditional societies where individual members are tightly bound by a single belief system, individuals are more likely to sacrifice their lives (as in the case of the martyr) for the greater good of the community, whereas fatalistic suicide occurs when traditional norms and belief systems operate as oppressive structures of regulation.

Durkheim suggests that modern societies are marked by a rise in egoistic and anomic suicides reflecting a breakdown in social bonds and traditional norms following certain social trends such as political apathy, hyper-individualism, the prevalence of nihilistic philosophies, and the widening of social choices at the same time that the norms and moral reference points on how we should live are loosened. Although Durkheim was making these observations over a hundred years ago, they remain pertinent to contemporary commentaries on the social causes of rising suicide rates. A central theme in his approach to the problem of social integration and regulation is the idea that associational forms of social organization are necessary to counter-balance such tendencies. This idea is re-emerging in social capital theory marking what Blaxter (2000) and Turner (2003) describe as a 'neo-Durkheimian' turn in social theory, which is discussed more fully under the application of structural functionalism to health in the following section.

Parsonian functionalism

For our present purpose, we now turn our attention to the development of structural functionalism (sometimes referred to simply as 'functionalism') as formulated in the work of the American sociologist, Talcott Parsons. Parsons is considered a central figure in the development of modern social theory and his work has left a deep imprint on the development of medical sociology. Influenced by the psychoanalytical theory of Freud, Parsons is interested in the motivations behind illness behaviour and how this is managed in the doctor–patient relationship (Turner 1992). However, Parsons' analytical framework extends beyond the therapeutic encounter to understanding the doctor–patient relationship in terms of the functional needs of society. Therefore, much of the commentary on Parsons' contribution to the sociology of health and illness has focused on his structural analysis of the illness experience. For Parsons, the structures of society (social roles, norms and values) are organized on the basis of its functional needs. In other words, they have a purpose and that purpose is to make society run smoothly. The core of his work is concerned with the problem of social order – how society reproduces and maintains an ordered structure or a state of balance between the different parts of the social system. Unlike the social interactionist theorists discussed in Chapter 3, Parsons does not take the micro-level of individuals interacting with one another as the basic unit of analysis in the study of society. Instead, his work is concerned with the large-scale structural components of the social system and its functional imperatives, including the necessity to maintain social order. It is important to note, however, that Parsons does not dismiss the importance of the micro-level of social interaction; his seminal work *The Social System* (1951), for example, is based on the interactions between doctors and patients in a Boston hospital. However, in understanding the relationship between actors and social structures, Parsons is interested in the way that people are socialized into the norms and values of a given social system and appropriate social roles.

Parsons is not just concerned with explaining individual action but with how that action may be determined by the way the social environment is organized. This idea is developed in his 'action system theory'. In this schema, there are four interrelated action systems – the social, cultural, behavioural and personality systems. The 'social system' consists of four subsystems (Parsons was very fond of the number four), which perform different but interrelated functions in maintaining the system as a whole. The economy serves the function of adapting the external environment to the needs of society through the organization of labour, production and distribution. The political system performs the function of defining common goals and mobilizing society to that end. The socialization system consists of the main institutions for socializing actors into the dominant norms, values and expectations of society, such as the family and educational system. The societal community serves the function of integrating and regulating the other components of the social system through formal legal codes and informal social control (Layder 1994, Ritzer and Goodman 2003). Balance between the various sub-systems of the social system, which is necessary for social stability, is achieved through the exchange of various forms of what Parsons calls 'symbolic media', such as money in the economy, power in the political system and influence and commitment in the societal community and socialization systems, respectively. The 'cultural system' refers to the stock of resources (knowledge, ideas and shared symbols such as language) available within a given society that individuals draw on to help them make sense of their interactions with others. The cultural system is embodied in the norms and values of the social system and the orientations and motivations of individual actors. For Parsons, the 'behavioural organism' (the body) is shaped in interaction with the social environment through processes of learning and socialization, as is the 'personality system' (see Ritzer and Goodman 2003 for a more detailed discussion).

Parsons, therefore, is best described as a macro-theorist in that he understands large-scale social and cultural systems as exerting a determining influence on individual motivations and behaviours. When compared to Marxist theory in the next chapter, which also offers an overarching theory of society, structural functionalism ignores the role that material factors, such as money and power, play in the way that the social system is structured. Moreover, the role that core values and norms play in terms of social integration is seen as operating outside of material interests. But what concerns us here is the emphasis that Parsons places on socialization and social control as mechanisms for maintaining social stability. As Ritzer and Goodman (2003) note, Parsons' overarching concern with social order and the assumptions that he makes about the passivity of social actors in his strong version of socialization theory (the idea that people internalize norms, values and role expectations) have become major targets of criticism of his work.

Having outlined the key ingredients of Parsons' complex theoretical framework, we go on to look more closely at how he develops these insights in relation to healthcare, particularly his analytical model of the sick role (1951) in explaining key features of the doctor–patient relationship, and how he links these to the wider system problem of social stability.

Applications to understandings of health

The neo-Durkheimian turn and social capital theory

Since the mid-1990s there has been a growing literature linking social capital to a variety of outcomes including better health. In this section, we are particularly concerned with tracing the 'neo-Durkheimian' thread in the way the concept of social capital is applied in understanding the social determinants of health. As is often the case with other classical theories presented in this book, we find only a cursory mention to Durkheim in the contemporary research field on social capital and health, which also largely ignores his work on suicide. However, the link between the classical theoretical precepts outlined in the previous section is suggested by the way that social capital is used as an umbrella term encapsulating the ideas of social integration, social cohesion and social support (Almedom 2005). The key bodies of work that have shaped social capital theory in the field of health research are Robert Putnam's *Bowling Alone: The Collapse and Revival of American Community* (2000) and Richard Wilkinson's *Unhealthy Societies: The Afflictions of Inequality* (1996), and the application of their theories in the much-cited research of Kawachi *et al.* (1997, 1999a). This body of work may be interpreted as neo-Durkheimian in the sense that social capital is understood as a property of social structures and social relationships whose function is to promote social support through norms and values of trust and reciprocity and that, at the same time, regulate deviant behaviour. This conceptualization of social capital proves to be the major point of contention in Marxist materialist analyses in which the link between social inequalities and health inequalities is bound up with the social relations of production in capitalist societies (Muntaner and Lynch 1999, Navarro 2002; see also Chapter 2). We will now consider how social capital theory is applied to understanding the social determinants of health by exploring the following:

- Definitions of social capital based on its relational dimensions (emphasizing the norms and values that connect people to one another) and its material dimensions (emphasizing social capital as a resource that is determined by an individual's socio-economic or class position);
- How the links between social capital and health outcomes are conceptualized in the key social capital literature, and finally;
- Empirical evidence of the link between social capital and health outcomes.

Defining social capital: The relational dimension

The relational dimension of social capital includes norms, values, social networks, trust and reciprocity, social integration, social cohesion and social support. The core elements of the relational definition are encapsulated in Putnam's (1995, 2000) theory of social capital, which dominates the health research literature (Moore *et al.* 2005), and these may be summarized in the following way:

a) Membership of social groups or networks (personal or primary social networks such as family, friends, neighbours, co-workers; and secondary, formal networks such as voluntary organizations and statutory organizations).
b) The norms and values that confer obligations and benefits on individual members of the social network (such as trust, reciprocity, access to strategic resources, sense of belonging and social control).
c) The outcomes (and function) of social capital (such as social support, civic participation, social cohesion).

Putnam's (1993) original thesis is based on the idea that social capital as a measure of civic participation is a prerequisite to democratic culture, effective political governance and economic development. In 'Bowling Alone' (1995), he equates the demise in the American sense of community with a perceived loss of quality of life. The public health literature draws on Putnam's concept of social capital as a 'civic' property of communities, which he defines as '...features of social organization such as networks, norms, and social trust that facilitate action and cooperation for mutual benefit' (1995: 67). An important feature of Putnam's definition of social capital is that he understands it as a collective property of society rather than as a property of individuals. The 'stock' of social capital available in a given community is measured by a number of predictive indicators, including membership in voluntary organizations (social capital networks), democratic participation (newspaper consumption, voting patterns and preferences) and expressions of interpersonal trust and reciprocity and institutional trust (social capital values). Putnam also identifies different forms of social capital. Bonding social capital refers to primary social groups and informal social networks such as family, kin and friendship networks. Strong ties amongst people who share core beliefs, which promote shared values, mutual trust and norms of reciprocity, typically characterize this kind of network. As well as contributing to an individual's sense of self-worth, this type of network is also a source of informal social control. Bridging social capital refers to a looser network of both horizontal and vertical connections between heterogeneous groups, for example between different community/voluntary groups and between these groups and other organizations such as statutory agencies involved in decision–making about the distribution of public goods and services (Almedom 2005). While these secondary, formal institutional networks constitute weaker ties amongst members, they are usually more inclusive than bonding forms of social networks. This type of network promotes collective efficacy and collective decision-making through community and civic participation. There is a strong theoretical correlation here with Durkheim's distinction between mechanistic and organic forms of solidarity. Like Durkheim, Putnam does not argue that we should return to traditional forms of social cohesion, but create new forms of association that can adapt to contemporary social conditions. More recently, Szreter and Woolcock (2004: 655) draw a further distinction between the kind of relationships that define horizontal connections between people who are 'more or less equal in terms of their power and status' and those that 'connect people across explicit "vertical" power differentials', for example, when people are accessing resources from formal institutions such as healthcare. They refer to the latter as 'linking' social capital.

Defining social capital: The material dimension

Those theories that emphasise social capital as a 'public good' and identify social participation and engagement as the key features of social capital accumulation in society belong to the neo-Durkheimian turn. While

Putnam's work stands out in this respect, the concept of social capital is also traced to the work of sociologists James Coleman (1988) and Pierre Bourdieu. Bourdieu's theory of social capital is of particular interest to our discussion because many of the critiques of Putnam's theory point out that the *material* as opposed to the *relational* (the social relationships that form an individual's social ties) dimension of social capital is ignored (Portes 1998, Hawe and Shiell 2000), along with the potentially negative effects of social capital (Muntaner and Lynch 1999), which Bourdieu's theory addresses. More recently, some researchers suggest a productive synergy between Putnam's and Bourdieu's conceptualizations of social capital (Ziersch 2005, Carpiano 2006).

Bourdieu's theory suggests a material analysis – one that is concerned with social power and the question of how access to social capital as a resource is determined by wider socio-economic structures. Bourdieu defines social capital as 'the aggregate of the actual or potential resources which are linked to possession of a durable network of more or less institutionalized relationships of mutual acquaintance and recognition' (1986: 248). He links social capital to the cultural, social and economic dynamics of class formation and, therefore, to other forms of capital including economic capital and cultural capital (such as education). Social networks differ in the amount and transferability of social capital as a resource that individual members can mobilize. In other words, social capital is differently distributed in society and this reflects broader inequalities. Therefore, if Bourdieu's theory was integrated into social capital studies, social network analysis would not only be concerned with social support and social participation and engagement (as a civic measure) but also with the way that social networks can work exclusively by giving group members access to influence and material resources. As Ziersch (2005) argues, Bourdieu's understanding that social capital can serve to reproduce existing social inequalities questions the universal value attributed to social capital as a public good in the way Putnam and his followers assume.

Linking social capital to health outcomes

The basic hypothesis in the health research literature is that certain features of the social environment associated with social capital promote positive health. Wilkinson's (1996) seminal work explaining the relationship between income inequality and health inequality has stimulated considerable debate and research on the role that social capital plays in health outcomes. While the relationship between income inequality and health inequality is strongly supported by empirical evidence, the mechanisms by which income inequality impact on health are often disputed. We will see that political economists (Chapter 2) and critical realists (Chapter 5) have different interpretations. Wilkinson observes that the wealthiest countries are not necessarily the healthiest societies. He argues that there is a threshold beyond which the absolute wealth of a population no longer has a direct bearing on health in wealthy countries that have undergone an epidemiological shift in the burden of disease from acute, infectious diseases to chronic illnesses. Wealthy societies that show unequal outcomes for health also have the greatest income inequalities and are less socially cohesive. This leads Wilkinson to argue that social capital as a psychosocial pathway is the key mechanism that mediates the relationship between income inequality and health inequality. In other words, the amount of social capital an individual has will affect how that individual thinks, feels and behaves. He suggests that this is the case because in unequal societies there is less social cohesion and people's perceptions of social exclusion and sense of alienation serve to exclude them from the dominant ethos of a society. The psychosocial impact of exclusion (anxiety, feelings of hopelessness, anger and insecurity) leaves its mark on health both directly in terms of the impact of the social environment on the individual's immunity and indirectly in terms of health behaviours. In socially cohesive societies the social environment is a source of social support rather than a source of social instability that undermines supportive social networks and, hence, the well-being of the whole society.

The key question for health researchers then is *what does social capital tell us about the mechanisms by which income inequality impacts on health?* Drawing directly on the work of Putnam, the overarching hypothesis is that social capital in the form of voluntary association and the density (size and frequency of social interaction) of the network amongst these associations in the community is protective of health. Putnam's basic theoretical argument is that civic participation in associations creates trust and reciprocity necessary for the social fabric of a society, which, in turn, sustains social relationships that provide mutual support within the community. High levels of social capital are necessary so that people can act collectively to demand better government and more efficient services for the common good. Kawachi *et al.* (1997) found a strong statistical correlation between social capital and health across 39 US states. Following Putnam, they measure social capital in terms of levels of trust and membership of voluntary associations and argue that income inequality impacts on health negatively through the social capital variable. The mechanisms by which social capital affects health outcomes suggest a number of direct and indirect pathways. First, community social capital influences the health of individuals by providing social support, mutual respect and self-esteem. In communities with low stocks of social capital, a direct pathway linking social capital to health is the psychosocial stress caused by insufficient social networks, limited social participation and lack of community empowerment (Wilkinson 1996, Kawachi et al. 1999a, Kawachi and Kennedy 1999). Second, an indirect pathway is that communities with high stocks of social capital are more likely to collectively mobilize for better public services and amenities that are relevant to health (Kawachi et al. 1999a).

A Marxist materialist perspective (developed under the political economy approach in Chapter 2) argues that the social relations of production in capitalist society influence all aspects of life including health and well-being. From the point of view of a Marxist materialist critique, Muntaner and Lynch (1999) argue that social cohesion may well mask class relations within society, and they point out that the middle class generally has more resources to commit to their communities and public participation (also Altschuler et al. 2004). Furthermore, Cattell (2001) argues that network typologies (such as bonding and bridging) themselves may be describing class structures, while descriptions of the kind of resources available through networks may well be pointing to the processes involved in the production of health inequalities.

Assessing the evidence of the link between social capital and health outcomes

If we take the two basic hypotheses that emerge from Putnam's and Wilkinson's work – respectively, voluntary association and the density of community networks is protective of health, and social capital is an independent mediating variable linking income inequality and health inequality – we find contradictory evidence. Kawachi et al. (1997) found that higher levels of trust and higher levels of participation in social clubs and associations were linked to lower levels of mortality for most major causes of death. Kawachi et al. (1999) found that individuals living in states with a low stock of social capital reported higher levels of ill-health even after controlling for socio-economic status (income and education) and other individual risk factors such as access to healthcare, smoking and obesity. Expanding on this work, Veenstra (2000) did not find a strong statistical relationship between involvement in extended social networks such as clubs and associations and self-related health. He found that trust (in government, community, neighbours and identity groups) and its psychosocial components (sense of identity and commitment) were not significantly linked to self-related health after controlling for socio-economic status. He also found no direct relationship between civic participation and health and any tentative relationships disappeared once he controlled for socio-economic status. The only strong relationships that he found were between socio-economic status (income and education variables) and health.

Cooper *et al.*'s (1999 cited in Campbell 2000: 184) review of health survey data in England also found that material deprivation and socio-economic position had a stronger statistical correlation with adverse health than social capital indicators. However, this statistical relationship is weakened when variation in neighbourhood social capital is controlled suggesting that the context factors of community are important in the link between income inequality, social capital and health inequalities.

So, what do community-based studies on the role of social capital in economically deprived and socially excluded areas tell us? Again, the evidence is very mixed, but these studies paint a more complex picture. Some of the complexities of the association between social capital and health have been well documented at the individual level in studies of social support and social networks in deprived communities. The key hypothesis of these studies is that social supports in the form of primary and informal networks such as family, kin and neighbourhood and formal supports in terms of local services act as a buffer against the health impacts of poverty. These studies show that the structure and function of social networks as a source of social support depends on the social context and that within a given community these networks are not unambiguously supportive either at the individual level or in terms of the social fabric of the community (Campbell 2000, Cattell 2001, Kunitz 2004). We will return to these arguments in Chapter 2. There is strong evidence to support the link between socio-economic status and individual health outcomes and equally strong empirical evidence to support the link between area-based deprivation and high community levels of mortality and morbidity. However, there is very little research on how community context affects different resident groups (Stafford *et al.* 2005).

In terms of conceptual and operational clarity there is a need to distinguish between the different sources of social capital and its functions as a measure of the effects attributed to social capital (Portes 1998). Ziersch (2005) offers a clear operational definition that distinguishes between these two conceptualizations in order to examine the relationship between sources of social capital and their outcomes, and how the social process involved in the interaction between these two elements impacts on health:

> SC [social capital] is conceptualized as comprising: *infrastructure* (SCI) – the networks and values that facilitate access to resources; and *resources* (SCR) – the resources available through this infrastructure. (Ziersch 2005: 2119)

Ziersch's (2005: 2128) operational definition of social capital incorporates Bourdieu's conceptualization of social capital, which not only emphasizes '...the ties between people but also the "value" of these ties in terms of accruing resources'. He applies this conceptualization to a quantitative survey of two suburbs in West Adelaide, Australia. Ziersch's main findings are that within a community people will have access to different kinds of social networks depending on their socioeconomic status and that some types of social networks are more important for accessing the kind of resources that are protective of health. For example, he found that the informal networks and values associated with being better off also led to better social capital resources that were also linked to better health. However, in line with other studies (a community study by Baum *et al*. (2000) also conducted in Australia, and Veenstra's (2000) Canadian community survey), he found that formal social networks had no relationship to either self-reported mental or physical health. The psychosocial components of social capital resources in this study were respondents' feelings of acceptance, measured by the statement, 'I don't feel fully accepted as a member of [the area]', and the extent to which people felt in control of their lives. Feelings of acceptance were not linked to either mental or physical health, while an individual's sense of control was positively linked to mental health. In Ziersch's study this psychosocial component is linked to social support that directly arises from informal networks rather than from the civic actions that are linked to formal networks. People's perception of relative advantage were also included in the survey and respondents were asked to score their sense of advantage relative to others in the locality in terms of family life, achievements, money and material possessions, quality of life and so on (see Ziersch 2005: 2123 for a full list of indices for this variable). This variable was positively linked with income level and tenancy (whether people rent or own their homes), and indirectly with work status and education. Not surprisingly, those with better incomes, who owned their homes, were employed and had higher educational credentials were more likely to perceive themselves as relatively advantaged compared to others in their locality. These socio-economic factors are also linked with those elements of social capital that were positively associated with perceptions of relative advantage. While people's perceptions of relative advantage were directly related to mental health, this was only marginally so in relation to physical health.

The primary research that we use as examples to discuss the impact of social capital on health show very mixed and contradictory results (see also Almedom's (2005) review of the research linking social capital and mental health, as well as Hawe and Shiell's (2000) assessment of the literature on social capital and health promotion). The difficulty of assessing the primary evidence is compounded by theoretical and methodological differences within the literature. Primary studies draw on different theoretical definitions of social capital, which produce different indicators of social capital; these studies also follow different research designs and use different sampling techniques, sample sizes and units of analysis. Some studies are concerned with individual level analysis of social capital (Veenstra 2000, Ziersch 2005), others are concerned with measuring the effect of community or aggregate social capital on health (Kawachi *et al.* 1997), while others again are concerned with the contextual effect of community-level social capital or neighbourhood environment on individual health (Cattell 2001, Stafford *et al.* 2005).

Campbell (2000: 182) argues that the utility of social capital theory for understanding the social determinants of health and its usefulness for informing health policy and health interventions depends on research 'identifying measurable indicators of what constitutes a health-enabling community'. However, the empirical field remains dominated by statistical studies, and Almedom (2005) contends that the dearth of qualitative and ethnographical studies of social capital makes it particularly difficult to interpret the causal relationships between different variables produced by statistical data. He suggests that qualitative studies are necessary in order to contextualize and demonstrate the relevance of statistical evidence for policy and practice. While larger aggregate surveys of income inequality and health are more likely to capture significant statistical relationships, smaller scale qualitative studies have explanatory value in demonstrating the conceptual links between the cultural, relational and material aspects of social capital in mediating the relationship between poverty, social exclusion and health (see in particular Cattell 2001).

Applications to understandings of healthcare

Structural functionalism and healthcare: Developments and critiques

Having examined how the contemporary heirs of structural functionalism understand health and its determinants, we now move back in time to examine the seminal application of structural functionalism to the understanding of healthcare, specifically to the traditional doctor–patient relationship. The doctor–patient relationship is a central component of healthcare since doctors define the needs and treatment of patients, albeit increasingly in the context of healthcare management and governmental guidelines (see Chapter 2 for further discussion on the professional position of doctors). This relationship also demonstrates the links between the micro- and macro-politics of healthcare since it is bound up with public trust in medicine and the authority that is invested in professional values and expert knowledge. Parsons' theory of the 'sick role' is his enduring legacy to the sociology of medicine in terms of stimulating both a wealth of research and instructive criticisms. In this section we trace the shifts in research in professional–patient relationships under the following themes:

- The 'sick role' and its theoretical limitations in understanding professional–patient relationships;
- Illness experience and the challenge that chronic illness posits for Parsons' concept of the sick role;
- Patient-centred approaches to medical care and the shift away from paternalistic healthcare relationships.

The 'sick role'

Parsons, in *The Social System* (1951: 430), wrote that '...from the point of view of the functioning of the social system, too low a general level of health, too high an incidence of illness, is dysfunctional: this is in the first instance because illness incapacitates the effective perfor-mance of social roles'. Here we see how Parsons defines health in terms of our ability to function normally and to fulfil our role obligations. Illness, therefore, is not simply a biological category but it has a social dimension. Parsons understands that there is degree of motivation attached to all forms of illness, in the sense that consciously or subcon-sciously we may be motivated to withdraw from our social roles and obligations, for example when we are unable to cope with the stresses of everyday life. Hence, he defines illness as a potential form of social deviance, which requires some mechanism of control and regulation. Parsons developed the analytical model of the 'sick role' to explain how society regulates illness behaviour through a system that makes explicit social expectations concerning individual behaviour. The sick role is a particular kind of 'status role' that the sick person can tem-porarily occupy in order to recuperate from illness free from the obliga-tions of their everyday social roles. Doctors are the gatekeepers of the sick role: by certifying an illness the doctor sanctions the sick role and, therefore, controls the private motivations of individuals to avoid social responsibilities such as work. The sick role orientates both patients and doctors towards mutual expectations about their respec-tive roles. These roles are governed by a set of rights and duties, which the doctor controls ultimately. The sick person has a right to be exempt from the expectations of their everyday social roles and from responsi-bility or blame for their illness on condition that they seek out com-petent healthcare and comply with the doctor's orders. The doctor, on the other hand, is obliged to give competent care and to be guided by the patient's best interest.

The rights acquired by doctors in their professional role stem from their expertise and their professional commitment of service to the community over self-interest. The interaction between doctors and patients is guided by what Parsons terms 'pattern variables', which determine the parameters of interaction that shape role expectations. The doctor must not relate to patients in terms of particular criteria (e.g., dealing with patients in specific ways because they belong to a particular social category) or become emotionally attached (the ideal of professionalism); instead, the doctor must treat all patients equally on the basis of their illness (the principle of universalism). Here we see how the sick role is conceived by Parsons as a rule-bound social sys-tem that is governed by social roles, role expectations and a system of guiding values. Parsons' characterization of the relationship between doctor and patient as consensual mirrors his macro-theory of society, which is based on the idea of a harmonious fit between the functional needs of society and its institutional structures (systems integration) and a high level of social integration where people adhere to a core set of norms and values to guide their actions with one another.

The theoretical limitations of the 'sick role'

While Parsons emphasizes that his theory of the sick role is based on an 'ideal type' (an analytical construct that identifies the most important general features of the doctor–patient relationship, but does not necessarily describe all actual instances of that relationship) his characterization of the doctor–patient relationship as one that is based on cooperation and mutual benefit has been subject to much critique, as has his depiction of the ideal patient as passive and compliant in deferring to the expertise of the doctor. An overarching critique of functionalist theory is that it ignores structural relations of power in society. In the context of the doctor–patient relationship this blinkers Parsons to the way that structural relations of power such as class, gender or ethnicity impacts on the illness experience and mediates the relationship between health professionals and patients. Moreover, as a consensus theorist, he sees the power structures of society as a legitimate means of maintaining social order, therefore, the power of the medical profession as an agent of social control is understood in Parsons' terms as a functional prerequisite of society. By emphasizing the norms and values that structure the doctor–patient relationship, Parsons neglects the material interests of such a powerful interest group and the role that biomedical ideology plays in the maintenance of power relations (Freidson 1986). The currency of this Parsonian model of the doctor–patient relationship perhaps lies less with its explanatory power than in the way that it measures up to a commonsensical view of the cultural power of medicine, which is the viewpoint that the power imbalance between doctor and patient is inevitable by virtue of the doctor's technical expertise and the vulnerability of patients who are reliant on the doctor's advice and willingness to act on their behalf so that they can access health resources.

Parsons' theory of the sick role has given rise to a significant body of empirical studies on the doctor–patient relationship and illness behaviour, primarily concerned with understanding patient compliance. However, the sick role theory (defined as doctor-centred) has been overtaken by new analytical perspectives that explore how the doctor–patient relationship mediates, if not mirrors, broader relations of power and knowledge, for example in feminist critiques of how women are constructed in healthcare encounters (see Chapter 6). Similarly, studies on illness behaviour have begun to problematize the notion of the passive patient, as well as exploring the contextual determinants of behaviour. There is not space here to offer a review of these diverse developments; instead, we will focus on the shift from a focus on illness behaviour to illness experience (Lawton 2003), which arose, in part, from the limitations of Parsons' sick role theory for understanding chronic illness, and the shift in healthcare philosophies from doctor-centred to patient-centred approaches.

Illness experience and the challenge of chronic illness

One of the major critiques of Parsons' sick role theory is that it assumes an episodic view of illness as acute, temporary and potentially curable. The burgeoning chronic illness research literature that began to emerge in the 1980s represents a concern with lay knowledge and subjective experience as part of a growing sociological critique of the dominance of biomedicine. In this sense, the new research interest is seen as part of a wider cultural shift, which Bury (2001: 265) describes as '…the loosening of the authority of the "grand narratives" of science and medicine in the ordering of everyday experience'. Chronic diseases by definition are long-standing debilitating illnesses that cannot be cured and, therefore, challenge medical certainty and the cultural authority of medicine invested in the quest for cure. The growing body of empirical studies and conceptual work on people's experience of chronic illness challenge the underlying theoretical and practical premises of Parsons' theory which, as May et al. (2006: 1024) note, is echoed more widely in '…structural and policy shifts in the organization of health care'. This is most notable in changing philosophies of health that emphasize patient-centred therapeutic approaches and holistic models of care promoted in particular professional contexts such as nursing, general practice and occupational therapy; the emerging policy ideology of the patient as discerning customer; and the promotion of the self-care ethic in the new drive towards preventative strategies and health promotion (see also Chapter 4 for a more critical reading of these trends).

There are many aspects of the chronic illness experience that challenge the assumptions underlining Parsons characterization of the doctor–patient relationship and his theory of the sick role. For example, the premise that access to the sick role is universal and that those who enter the sick role are exempt from personal responsibility or blame for their condition is challenged by what Conrad (2004a: 130) refers to as 'contested illnesses' or 'elusive illnesses' that appear to defy organic explanations and, therefore, are 'biomedically invisible' (Barker 2004: 134).[1] For example, in a study involving the illness narratives of 30 Finnish women who suffered back pain, Lillrank (2003) found that their sense of self was threatened by the medical disparagement that the women encountered, and that the moral core of these women's self-narrative accounts was the stigmatizing effect of that experience. For psychiatrist and social anthropologist Arthur Kleinman, chronic illness raises the spectre of moral experience in contemporary life and challenges the strict boundary between lay knowledge and technical expertise in the quest for a humanistic approach to healthcare (1988, also Kleinman and Seeman 2000). This challenges Parsons idealization of the passive patient who defers to the doctor's expert and superior knowledge and the assumption that the unequal power relationship between doctor and patient is necessarily a functional imperative of a wider system-based need, which is underscored by relations of trust and mutual benefit. It also challenges the privilege status afforded to technical knowledge and foregrounds the potential for conflict to emerge between experiential understandings of illness grounded in everyday explanatory frameworks and expert definitions based on technical know-how and theoretical models. For example, chronically ill people are often very knowledgeable about medical treatments, pharmacological and technological advances in medical science, alternative therapies and environmental risks. Furthermore, in negotiating therapeutic regimes patients may reject the 'sick role' duties and the 'medical logic' of compliance for a 'social logic', which involves trade-offs that balance the demands of daily life with medical regimes (Conrad 2004b). Parsons view of the traditional doctor–patient relationship is incapable of grasping the possibility of conflict between the doctor's belief system, which informs clinical decision-making and the values and beliefs that the patient brings to the medical encounter.

---

[1] There is much research to support this observation from the patient's perspective and experience of what has become defined as 'functional somatic syndromes', such as Fibromyalgia Syndrome (FMS), Chronic Fatigue Syndrome (CFS) or Myalgic Encephalomyelitis (ME), Premenstrual Syndrome (PMS), Irritable Bowel Syndrome (IRB) and others.

The conceptual themes running through the research on the experience of chronic illness include the loss of identity experienced in the face of profound uncertainty when people can no longer rely on what Kleinman (1988: 45) aptly describes as the 'the fidelity of [their] bodies'. For the chronically ill person, health or normal bodily processes and daily activities can no longer be taken for granted. The defining feature of chronic illness is less about biophysical changes than it is about what researchers have variously described as a 'loss of self' (Charmaz 1983), 'social death' (Kleinman 1988) and 'biographical disruption' (Bury 1982, discussed in Chapter 3). Another theme is the impact of chronic illness on daily living and social interactions, including the loss of social and economic status, and the impact that this has on other family members who are cast in the carer's role (Charmaz 2000). Yet another theme is the coping strategies that people with chronic illness develop in actively creating meaningful lives in the context of managing felt and enacted stigma (Scambler and Hopkins 1986), and in mobilizing resources to help them to cope (Pierret 2003 citing Anderson and Bury 1988). These studies on chronic illness experience, which are further explored in Chapter 3, expand, albeit in a more critical fashion, Parsons original insight that illness has a strong social dimension.

Patient-centred approaches to medical care

In the context of our current discussion on the limitations of the Parsonian model, it will suffice to note that the shift in research focus from illness behaviour to illness experience represents an emerging trend in health research. This reconceptualizes the boundaries between lay/patient knowledge and expert knowledge and understands the therapeutic encounter as a negotiation between the different explanatory frameworks that health professionals and patients or primary caregivers draw on to explain the meaning of illness and shared decision-making about treatment. For example, in the social scientific literature on doctor–patient relationships, particularly in the area of general medical practice, there has been a notable shift away from patient compliance studies to an emphasis on patient-centred models of interaction and shared decision-making (Ainsworth-Vaughn 1998, Bensing et al. 2000, Mead and Bower 2000, Roter 2000 cited in Hyde et al. 2004: 145; see also the professional-practice based-text, Stewart et al. 2003). These studies represent two critical lines of departure from the assumptions that underlie Parsons' functionalist theory. At the micro-level of the doctor–patient encounter, Parsons' key blind spot is that he ignores the possibility of conflict between the doctor's belief system, which informs clinical decision-making, and the values and beliefs that the patient brings to the medical encounter. At the macro-level, Parsons presents medical hegemony as a functional imperative of the social system to maintain social order. However, public trust underlying medical authority in the doctor–patient relationship can no longer be assumed. The ideal type of patient once assumed to be passive, deferent and compliant in medical encounters is now expected to be responsible for her health and knowledgeable (see Chapter 4 for a poststructuralist critique of the 'self-responsibilization' of health). For example, expert knowledge is more widely available through electronic media and new forms of virtual communities exist for the dissemination of competing expert information (Nettleton 2004) and the sharing of healthcare and illness experiences.[2]

While many studies contend that there is a decisive shift away from paternalistic healthcare relationships, there are many contingencies at play in terms of what patients expect and need in therapeutic encounters. Notwithstanding the cultural differences in relation to how both patients and doctors view their respective roles, not all patients at all times want to have responsibility for decision-making, which is not the same as saying that patients do not want information relevant to their diagnosis and treatment. The kind of contingencies that come into play in terms of patients' preferences for a more active or passive role in treatment decisions include social factors such as age, gender or cultural background, as well as individual factors such as the severity of the patient's condition, their emotional needs and the extent to which taking responsibility for treatment is an additional and unwelcome burden (Coulter and Fitzpatrick 2000). Coulter and Fitzpatrick (2000) also note that one of the implications of shifting decision-making towards the consumer is the resource implication that this places on healthcare in terms of patients' rising expectations. Of course there are many factors that drive an ever-expanding healthcare market, not least, as Coulter and Fitzpatrick observe, the ideological emphasis of biomedicine on the benefits as opposed to the risks of treatment.

---

[2] An interesting web-based research initiative is the DIPEx project based on patients' personal experiences of illness and healthcare (www.dipex.org).

Conclusion and new directions for healthcare

This chapter addressed the contribution of structural functionalism to a sociological understanding of health and healthcare. We have noted that structural functionalism is a body of theory that is primarily concerned with explicating the macro-structures of society and that the major integrating idea linking the classical work of Durkheim to Parsons is the importance of social integration and regulation to the functioning of society as a cohesive whole. The two main criticisms of structural functionalism linking the classical work of Durkheim to Parsons' theory of social action are: (a) social life is primarily understood in terms of norms and values to the neglect of material aspects of the social world, and (b) social structures in the form of norms and values determine social action, which leaves no room for human agency or understanding social action in the context of how people make sense of the experiences of their everyday lives (see Chapter 3). These critiques re-emerge in the debate on social capital theory and the explanatory value of the neo-Durkheimian turn, particularly in relation to the question about what aspect of the social context of people's lives influences health outcomes, and how the relationship between the micro- and macro-levels of the social context can be re-theorized in order to explain the complex pathways of health and illness. As our discussion shows, social capital is a complex and multifaceted concept that is subject to different and competing theoretical expositions, yielding contradictory empirical evidence and competing understandings about the mechanisms by which the stock of social capital may influence population health. Furthermore, there are no strong claims arising from the primary data on social capital that a direct correlation exists between social cohesion (as an outcome measure of social capital) and health equality.

Social capital is often viewed as synonymous with social cohesion. In part, at least, this can be explained by the way in which social capital has been popularized by a wider political discourse and infused with sometimes competing ideological investments in the ideal of community and voluntarism (the principle of relying on the voluntary action of community members instead of the state) as a panacea against the modern ills of individualism and anomie (Portes 1998, Hawe and Shiell 2000, Navarro 2002). Muntaner and Lynch (1999: 71) caution against the naivety of assuming that social cohesion is a cure-all for health inequalities. Indeed, they argue that such a political analysis harbours the risk that responsibility for health will be transferred to those working-class

communities with the least resources to build social capital leaving '...
untouched more fundamental economic and political relations'.
As Cattell (2001) argues, material deprivation and social exclusion are
both barriers to social inclusion and have a direct bearing on health.
Hawe and Shiell (2000) suggest that contrary to the neo-Durkheimian
emphasis on social capital found in Putnam's political theory, Bourdieu's
sociological theory may be more relevant to unravelling the contextual
complexities of communities. As Campbell (2000) points out, policy
makers are often unaware of the level of community resources or how
different community members access those resources. In relation to the
latter point, the reader may be reminded that the central point that
Bourdieu brings to social capital theory is that the capacity of individuals
to mobilize resources that are beneficial for health largely depends on
the broader structures of (in)equality. Small-scale, qualitative community studies of social capital and social networks also show that the idealization of community is often contrary to everyday experiences and that
cohesive communities are just as likely to be intolerant of difference,
which may be detrimental to an individual's health in terms of accessing
various resources and supports (Baum 1999). Indeed, there is a strong
rationale emerging in the research literature for more qualitative community-based studies to better understand the relational and material
dimensions of social capital and how these mediate, directly or indirectly, health outcomes.

Parsons' analytical model of the sick role is a staple in illness behaviour and doctor–patient relationship studies in what we might broadly
term social science research applied to medicine. The importance of
Parsons' work lies in its identification of the fact that being sick is not
simply a matter of biology – it also has profound social consequences for
both the individual and society. As such, notwithstanding all the criticisms, it has generated a large number of studies on professional–patient
relationships including instructive critiques. However, as discussed
earlier, structural functionalism has been challenged because it no
longer would appear to have explanatory power to address the current
realties of healthcare. Current debates about the extent to which the
professional dominance of medicine is in decline (see Chapter 2 on the
'proletarianization' of medicine) and concerns about the limits of biomedicine, particularly in the context of the growing problem of chronic
illness, directly challenge Parsons' structural analysis of the illness experience and professional dominance. Indeed, changing healthcare
philosophies and policies have recast the doctor–patient relationship
from a Parsonian consensual model to a negotiative model (Mead and

Bower 2000), which is reflected by new research agendas and theoretical developments on patient-centred models of communication, patient empowerment and the role of experiential knowledge as a legitimate source of authority in therapeutic decision-making and policy decisions about the governance of healthcare. We note that the shift in concern from health behaviours to illness experiences and the emphasis on lay knowledge offer a point of contrast to Parsons' theory of the sick role and the pre-eminence that his theory affords to the medical profession and expert knowledge. Following on from critiques of Parsons' sick role theory and the authority he invests in the medical profession by virtue of the functional role that it performs, new lines of enquiry are opening up that are further explored in various chapters in the book. If we see the burgeoning field of empirical studies on the lay experience of illness as a counter development to and shift away from a Parsonian focus on illness behaviour and macro-theoretical formulations, then it is important to ask in what way do these studies contribute to the key sociological concerns of social structure, social action and power relations? Chapter 3 deals further with the question of the problem of integrating micro- and macro-perspectives in accommodating agency while addressing the underlying structural conditions of healthcare encounters. Another line of enquiry is concerned more explicitly with the social power that derives from doctors' control of healthcare and the various challenges that the authority of medicine now encounters in the face of growing consumerism within healthcare, declining trust in medical authority and new strategies of healthcare governance (see Chapters 2 and 4). Undoubtedly, new research will begin to take shape around what Lupton (1997) sees as emerging dichotomies between paternalism and patient empowerment, expert and experiential knowledge and consumerism and medical authority.

CHAPTER 2

Political Economy Theory, Health and Healthcare

Introduction

In this chapter we explore the main tenets of the political economy perspective and its application to understandings of health and healthcare. The political economy perspective was most fully developed in the writings of Karl Marx who emphasized economic and class relations as the basic defining structure of society. In the first part of this chapter, we will elaborate the main features of the political economy approach. One of the primary contributions of the political economy perspective to the understanding of health is in foregrounding the impact of socio-economic conditions on the health of individuals and populations. Political economy theorists seek to show how differences in class relations in the labour market cause differences in health outcomes for different socio-economic groups. Evidence to support the claim of differential life expectancy by class was available during Marx's lifetime in Victorian England (Chadwick 1842) as it is today (Lynch *et al.* 2004, Marmot 2005, Bejakel and Goldblatt 2006, Wilkinson and Pickett 2006). In the second part of this chapter, we examine contemporary research on inequalities in health in order to critically appraise the political economy approach.

The political economy perspective has also been extremely influential in critiquing the direction of contemporary healthcare systems in globalizing capitalist economies. The primary critique arsing from political economy understandings of healthcare is that, under capitalism, healthcare has become a commodity which is bought and sold through the system of the market which creates inequalities in access to healthcare. Political economists argue that there is a fundamental contradiction between the pursuit of profit and the pursuit of health (Doyal with

36

Pennel 1979: 44). In applying this approach to understandings of healthcare in the second part of this chapter, we will focus on changes in the employment conditions of healthcare workers. We will review the impact of capitalism – especially the increased privatization and corporatization of healthcare services – on the work of healthcare professions. In particular, we will evaluate the evidence for the political economy inspired theory of the 'proletarianization', or downgrading, of the medical profession and medical work.

Principles of political economy

The influence of a political economy understanding of society is evident in many academic disciplines including Economics, Philosophy and Political Science and has also been the source of inspiration for socialist political movements. This is, in part, due to the fact that the principal originator of the political economy approach, Karl Marx (1818–1883), was himself an interdisciplinary thinker for whom the objective of social theory was to provoke social change. As a means of introducing Marx's writings, we will focus on three central themes which are core to the political economy approach. These are Marx's emphasis on the role of structure, particularly economic structures, in affecting wider aspects of society; the contradictions of the capitalist system which Marx believed would lead to crisis, conflict and inevitable change; and, finally, a materialist concept of change in industrialized societies.

> Men [sic] make their own history, but they do not make it just as they please, they do not make it under circumstances chosen by themselves, but under circumstances directly found, given and transmitted from the past. (Marx [1852] 1954: 10)

Marx advanced a theory of society that held that whilst individuals have choices, these choices are limited by the society in which they live – or, more specifically, by the economy in which they live. Marx was writing during the time of the development of industrializing capitalist societies. Marx believed that the way in which the production of goods and services is organized is fundamental to understanding the structure of society and the relations of individuals to one another within that society. He argued that the economy created an *infrastructure* that formed the foundation for other institutions such as religion, the family and systems of education, which he referred to as a *super-structure*. The nature of the superstructure depended upon that of the infrastructure. Marx held that in capitalist economies, the other influential institutions in society, such as the political classes, religious hierarchies and medical and legal elites, gain their power in society by their alliance with the capitalist classes, namely those who own and control the means of production. The means of production in industrializing capitalist societies was defined as the raw materials and instruments (machines and factories) necessary for production. Private ownership of the means of production was for Marx the crucial element leading to the division of society into unequal economic classes (Morrison 2006). In capitalist societies, wider social structures reflect and reinforce the ideals and values of the capitalist classes and they act to protect one another. Marx's emphasis on the power of structures in society to shape people's lives was, in part, a response to the common belief at the time (and now) that being poor is one's own fault. Marx believed this to be a form of 'false consciousness' whereby *individuals* are blamed for social problems, such as unemployment, illiteracy and ill-health, which are, instead, problems arising from the economic system in which they live, most notably the hierarchal and exploitative labour relations of capitalist society. However, Marx's writings did not deny agency or the possibility of individuals to exact change in their circumstances (see further below). His concept of 'praxis' was a political idea referring to the transformative powers of human agency through the radicalization of class consciousness (Delanty 2005: 68). Marx insisted that the point was not just to study the world but also to change it ([1888] 1974). We return to these Marxist ideas in Chapter 5 on critical realism.

Marx demonstrated how capitalist production is organized around fundamental system contradictions which strain capitalist economies. The central contradiction for Marx resides in the class conflict between a small group of people who own the resources for production – the manufacturing industries and other enterprises (the capitalist class) and those who, in order to survive, sell their labour to earn a living (the proletariat). The capitalist system implies an inevitable contradiction between these two groups, according to Marx, because the capitalist class must always seek to maximize profits by minimizing costs (labour costs), whereas the labourers seek wages to be as high as possible. Furthermore, the capitalist system creates a sense of 'alienation' amongst the workers – a sense of isolation due to their relative powerlessness over the organization and products of their labour.

Alienation is essentially the result of the exploitative labour relations endemic to the capitalist system. It is the process by which workers lose control over their labour (which becomes abstracted into a wage) and the self-defining characteristics of their labouring activity. Labour was essential for Marx, in terms of how it formed the basis for individuals to create self-identity and connections to a broader community (Morrison 2006).

Marx believed that these contradictions inherent to capitalism would eventually lead to a heightened class consciousness or shared sense of awareness of exploitation amongst the proletariat or working classes and that this, in turn, would generate class conflict leading to revolutionary social change. Class consciousness and class conflict are regarded in Marxist terms as inherent parts of capitalist societies. Although many current social theorists (e.g., Holton and Turner 1989, Beck 1992, Lash and Urry 1994) argue that the model of class divisions as advanced in Marxism has become weakened and paradoxically more complex – for example the original two-class model is now seen by many commentators as simplistic because of the emergence of a strong middle class, and significant differences within the ruling and working classes have also been identified – the concept of class-based inequality remains a central issue across the social sciences.

To deal with this complexity, many social science researchers have tended to turn to Max Weber ([1922: 120–123] 1978) rather than Marx for their definition of class. In following Weber, they use the criterion of 'life chances' rather than relations of production to develop class categories, combining occupations whose members have similar sources and levels of income, amounts of job security and chances of economic advancement and who have a similar location within systems of authority and control within the workplace and, hence, similar levels of autonomy. The US researchers tend to use a combination of income and education to act as a measure of social class-based differences in society, whereas British and Irish researchers tend to use scales derived from the Erikson–Goldthorpe Schema (E–G schema) (1992) such as the new official UK social class schema known as the National Statistics Socio-Economic Classification (NS-SEC) (for England, Scotland and Wales) (Office for National Statistics 2002). Broadly, the latter measures social class in terms of two main criteria: ownership of property (e.g., company, real estate) and employment conditions and relations (especially the amount of autonomy over one's work). However, while the (Weberian) life chances approach to the definition of class is the dominant one, as we shall see in Chapter 5, critical realist commentators have argued that the use of the Marxist definition of class is useful if we wish to examine the reasons behind the large and growing differences in life chances and health outcomes within Western societies.

Marx's ideas about revolutionary social transformation are based on a materialist conception of change. A materialist understanding of social transformation is one which attributes the causes of societal shifts to fundamental changes in the economic order – the ways in which people produce goods and services, as opposed to changing values and ideologies. This approach does not deny the salience of values and ideologies, but sees them as superstructural, whereas the material conditions are held as constituting the fundamental base on which ideas and values are founded. Marx envisaged that a proletariat revolution would lead to a socialist society that would end the deep divisions between the owners and labourers in capitalist economies and lead to a re-distribution of the products of labour more equally amongst all groups in society. Thus, for Marx, the huge schism between the rich and the poor is not inevitable and can be transformed by changing the organization of production in a society. Marx's materialist approach is sometimes critiqued as a form of 'economic determinism' that neglects the role of ideology in generating change. However, his emphasis on a materialist conceptualization of social change must be read in its historical context as an important critique of the dominant position of 'idealist philosophy', particularly that of Hegel, at the time of Marx's writing (Delanty 2005: 70). Idealist philosophy is a broad church of intellectual ideas which emphasizes that ideas are central to the ways in which material reality is defined and experienced. Thus, Marx's counter position was to insist on recognizing the powerful material forces that *shape* the world of ideas in philosophy, religion and culture in general. We return to this debate below when examining the relative importance of the material *versus* the psychological impact of socio-economic inequalities on our health.

Applications to understandings of health

The principal application of political economy theory to understanding health is in explaining the link between society (especially the economic and political structures of society) and patterns of morbidity and mortality. In particular, the political economy perspective highlights the existence of a causal relationship between inequalities in social class and inequalities in health. The Marxist concern for the health of the working classes developed through Marx's friendship with a fellow writer and activist, Frederich Engels. Engels' book entitled *The Condition of the Working Classes in England* ([1886] 1987) portrayed the ill-health and low life expectancy of workers compared with the bourgeoisie, along with the increasing tendency to suicide, and the very widespread drunkenness and 'sexual licence'. The latter, he remarked, were the only two pleasures the bourgeoisie has left the working classes. Engels concluded that the class differences between the working classes and bourgeoisie were such that the working class had virtually become a race wholly apart from the English bourgeoisie: 'The workers speak other dialects, have other thoughts and ideals, other customs and moral principles, a different religion and other politics than those of the bourgeoisie' (Engels [1886] 1987: 162). [Unsurprising, given many of them were not English at all but Irish immigrants to Manchester!] Another landmark study of the time was Edwin Chadwick's *Report of an Enquiry into the Sanitary Conditions of the Labouring Population of Great Britain* (1842). Chadwick, a public health pioneer, described how poverty and poor living environments in Victorian England, such as filth in the air, water, soil and surroundings, were major factors in the spread of disease, and Chadwick's study hastened the Public Health Act (1848) in Great Britain which formally linked health with socio-economic conditions.

Social class and health in contemporary societies

The relationship between social class and health – namely the lower your place in the social-class scale, the worse is likely to be your health status – has remained a remarkably stable empirical observation to the present day. In contemporary terms, there is an average difference of between 5 and 7 years in the life expectancy of those in the higher socio-economic classes and those in the lowest across many Western developed societies. The obduracy of this fact remains regardless of how studies have measured social class. We turn now to these studies of inequalities in health in Western societies in order to critically explore the value and saliency of the political economy theory in explaining relationships between social class and health. The primary debates over explanations for inequalities in health are:

- Materialist versus cultural/behavioural theories of health
- Neo-materialist versus psychosocial theories of health
- The life course approach.

Materialist versus cultural/behavioural theories of health

The so-called Black Report in the United Kingdom (Townsend *et al.* 1992) was a landmark study in re-launching the polemic on inequalities in health in post-war Britain. It was particularly controversial because it documented the persistence of health inequalities in a relatively affluent society in which standards of living, housing and sanitation, and access to healthcare had all improved. However, even though life expectancy was rising overall for the population, inequalities in life expectancy, as well as morbidity more broadly, had persisted. Four key explanations were explored in the Black Report to account for social-class patterns in health. These were the artefact explanation (health inequalities are an outcome of statistical processes), the social selection explanation (health inequalities determine economic inequalities not *vice versa*), cultural/behavioural explanations (health inequalities are an outcome of differing cultural attitudes to health and health behaviours) and materialist/structuralist explanation, which is derived from the political economy theory (health inequalities are an outcome of economic and associated socio-structural factors).

The Black Report concluded that the materialist/structuralist explanation offered the most plausible explanation of the way in which social class affects physical bodies, emphasizing the role of low income, unemployment, poor housing, poor communities and exposure to hazards in explaining the poorer health of individuals in the lower social classes relative to those in the higher social classes. The report rejected what Macintyre (1997) refers to as a 'hard' version of the cultural behavioural thesis that observable class differences are caused by health damaging behaviours, which are freely chosen by individuals in different social classes. Marxist political economists identify this cultural-behavioural explanation as a form of false consciousness whereby the assumption of freedom to choose a healthy lifestyle may not correspond to people's experiences of the wider set of material and environmental factors that shape people's lives and the choices available to them. Political economists argue that this hard version of the cultural behavioural explanation leads to a regressive public policy agenda of blaming individuals for not having the 'common sense' or education in terms of health information to adopt healthy behaviours (e.g., in relation to diet, smoking, drinking and exercise), rather than a public policy that addresses the social circumstances which constrain individual choice. Nonetheless, the Black Report did acknowledge the relationship between adverse health behaviours and accepted what Macintyre (1997) refers to as a 'soft version' of the cultural/behavioural thesis which suggests that health damaging behaviours are differentially distributed across social classes and contribute to inequalities in health (Macintyre 1997: 727).

In recent times, increased efforts have been made to combine these theories rather than to distinguish them. Thus the scientific literature in inequalities in health draws together a literature which examines inequalities at structural (community and global level factors) as well as at individual level factors (propensity to smoke, take exercise) into a unified framework (Lohan 2007). For example, a model of health developed by Dahlgreen and Whitehead for the World Health Organization (WHO) in the early 1990s and used widely in health inequalities research represents the determinants of health as adjacent layers of influence, one over another (see Bejakel and Goldblatt 2006). Another fruitful way of bringing together the Marxist political economy concern with the socio-economic determinants of health and a concern with health behaviours as a structural component of people's lives rather than as a property of individual volition has been developed by drawing on the work of Pierre Bourdieu. Specifically, Bourdieu's (1979) concept of 'habitus' – meaning a socially influenced disposition to think or act in particular ways – is used in some health inequalities literature (e.g., Lynch *et al.* 1997, Popay *et al.* 1998, Fassin 2000, Robertson 2006a, 2006b) to describe how bodies become shaped through daily unconscious practices that are nonetheless related to social relations of class, gender and ethnicity operating in society (Lohan 2007). According to Scott (2006: 168), the acquisition of a habitus is a direct consequence of involvement in particular recurrent social relations – class conditions, gender conditions and so on, which are associated with the formation of specific bodily skills and capacities, such as ways of walking, eating and talking, systems of tastes, preferences, forms of classification, and numerous other tendencies and dispositions. By integrating a combination of the cultural/behavioural model, albeit from a more critical interpretation, and materialist explanations, social scientists attempt to account for how the systemic aspects of social structure become embodied in our everyday lives through everyday practices.

Neo-materialist versus psychosocial theories of health

Further debates have been launched in the 1990s and 2000s in relation to inequalities in health which continue to be framed by the importance of political economy understandings of health inequalities. One of the most important contemporary debates has been between the neo-materialist and psychosocial theories of inequalities in health. The neo-materialist argument refers to the ways in which individual level inequalities are often combined with contextual or environmental level factors that also affect health. It is this clustering of individual level inequalities (availability of private resources) and societal level inequalities (such as investment in the public infrastructures of education, transport, healthcare, availability of food, quality of housing) that gives rise to the term 'neo-materialist'. It suggests that 'the inequalities in an individual's access to opportunities and material goods as well as differential systematic lack of investment in physical infrastructure result in health inequalities' (Huynh et al. 2005: 889). For example, individuals who live in areas of pollution are more likely to reside in poor-quality housing and more likely to eat a poor diet (Davey Smith et al. 1994: 139–140). The clustering of disadvantage based around social class is also evidenced in area-based studies of health, which look at the relationship between spatial resources and health. The findings of these studies show that more affluent areas tend to be better resourced in terms of quality retail facilities especially for foodstuffs, better physical environment including recreational facilities, better public services and record lower rates of violence and crime which, in turn, affords better health status to the populations of those areas (Macintyre et al. 1993, Shaw et al. 2002, Cohen et al. 2003, Heymenn et al. 2006). For example, Shaw et al. (2002) identified the 15 worst and 13 best health areas of Britain using premature mortality rates (deaths under 65). The population of the worst area of Britain was over two-and-a-half-times more likely to die prematurely than those in the wealthier and better resourced areas.

Turning now to the psychosocial explanation, this may also be seen to operate at the context-/area-based level, but it draws particular attention to the *psychological* as opposed to the material effects of one's surroundings on one's health. The psychosocial model places primacy on the psychological impact of adverse psychosocial exposures, such as stress, hostility, hopelessness, loss of control or, collectively, 'misery' on health (Macleod and Davey Smith 2003: 565). Evidence for this explanation draws on how experiences of stressful conditions at work or at home, or the general feeling of low social status may directly or indirectly affect physical health, particularly heart disease (Adamson *et al.* 2006). The argument is that the impact of low income, poor housing and employment conditions is not just, or primarily, related to the presence or absence of individual/social resources but rather through the psychosocial impact of these factors on one's self-esteem and ability to connect with others. According to Bartley: 'in most of the psycho-social literature, the focus is on how feelings that arise because of inequality, domination or subordination, may directly affect biological processes' (2004: 80).

The argument is most clearly drawn out at a context level in the 'unequal incomes theory'. Authors such as Wilkinson (1996) and Kawachi *et al.* (1999) argue that socio-economic differences in a society (inequalities) can create psychosocial reactions that impact on people's self-esteem, their sense of trust and their sense of being connected to the society around them. This sense of being connected is also called 'social capital' (measured in terms of social networks/social involvement) in society. They propose that this, in turn, leads to unhealthy coping behaviours, such as excessive drinking and smoking, and poorer health status (see Chapter 1 for a fuller discussion of social capital theory). According to this thesis, it is not necessarily poverty in itself that is damaging to health; rather, it is *relative poverty* and how this affects one's perception of oneself in society. However, the impact of relative poverty on health thesis is also keenly contested in the health inequalities literature. It has provoked a systematic review of 98 aggregate and multi-level studies on this question. The review concluded that:

> …overall, there seems to be little support for the idea that income inequality is a major, generalizable determination of population health differences within or between rich countries. Income inequality, may, however, directly influence some health outcomes, such as homicide in some contexts. (Lynch *et al.* 2004: 5)

The review went on to bolster the materialist relationship between *low* income and health to say that:

> Despite little support for a direct effect of income inequality on health *per se*, reducing income inequality by raising the incomes of the most disadvantaged will improve their health, help reduce health inequalities, and generally improve population health. (Lynch *et al.* 2004: 5)

Thus far, we have highlighted the main differences in the psychosocial and neo-materialist understandings of health. However, they also have points in common. Let us begin with the theoretical links. Whilst the neo-materialist explanation is rooted in Marxist political economy theory and the psychosocial explanation is associated with functionalist (social capital) theories derived from Durkheim, there are notable theoretical overlaps. As mentioned in the first part of this chapter, the theme of alienation is central to Marxist theory. In particular, the link between the psychosocial impact of working conditions should be seen to have a clear overlap with Marxist theory, in which labour also had a spiritual dimension (Delanty 2005). Indeed, Marmot and Wilkinson (2001), in developing their psychosocial argument, make direct reference to Marx's (1942) writings on 'paleo-materialism' in which Marx describes the psychological effect of inequality. Therefore, it has been argued within Marxist theory that 'the "mind" and 'body' are not separate either/or categories, but are dialectically related to each other' (Yuill 2005: 133). Yuill argues that materialists should not:

> ....shy away from acknowledging the important role that emotions play in poor health as emotions are one of the ways in which poor material circumstances are experienced. Alienation theory provides that linkage between the material and the emotional with the material circumstances and negative emotions being bound up dialectically with each other. (2005: 139)

Thus, from a theoretical point of view, focusing on emotions and the psychological effects of poverty and inequality is not incompatible with a Marxist political economy approach. However, the relative importance of these factors on causing inequalities in health is empirically disputed in the inequalities in health literature. Whilst many authors (notably MacLeod and Davey Smith 2003, Lynch et al. 2004, Adamson et al. 2006) do not deny the relationship between 'misery' and poverty as outlined in the work of Wilkinson (1996), Kawachi et al. (1999) and Marmot and Wilkinson (2001), they reject the primacy of the psychological explanation implied in the psychosocial explanation and, in particular as noted above, the psychological effect of unequal incomes on health status (Lynch et al. 2004). Nonetheless, this empirical disagreement means that the hypothesis remains live in large-scale quantitative research. In addition, in common with Bartley (2004), we suggest that it opens up possibilities for further qualitative research, where the relationship between the emotional impact of material inequalities on health and well-being may be more apparent.

The life course approach

One final approach which tries to combine political economy perspectives with a broader range of explanations derived from diverse theoretical roots is the *life course approach*. A life course approach to understanding inequalities in health is not a new or different explanation to those already discussed. Rather, a life course approach incorporates elements of these explanations and specifically focuses on the ways in which factors that impact on health combine over time to cause ill-health. The life-course explanation suggests that an individual's health status at any given age for a given birth cohort reflects not only contemporary conditions but embodiment of prior life conditions from *in utero* onwards (Kawachi *et al.* 2002: 650). Three conceptual models which capture this life course approach can be identified in contemporary research: a critical period model, a pathway model and an accumulation model (Lohan 2007). A *critical period model* (also known as latent effects or latency model) (Ben-Shlomo and Kuh 2002, Kawachi *et al.* 2002) suggests that diseases which make a greater contribution to the socio-economic gradient in health have their origins in critical periods of development. Critical period models tend to focus on the role of early life adversity, highlighting embryonic, infant and childhood periods (such as, Barker's (1998) foetal programming hypothesis) as major influences on disease risk in adulthood. The *pathway model* focuses on how the early life environment sets individuals onto life trajectories which have implications for health. For example, how childhood disadvantage may restrict educational opportunities and which may, in turn, restrict employment opportunities and health-related behaviours in later life. The *accumulation* or cumulative effects *model* suggests that the intensity or duration of exposure to unfavourable environments at different life stages has a cumulative or 'chain' adverse effect on health. According to this model, poor circumstances throughout life confer the greatest risk of poor health in adulthood. However, according to this model also, poor circumstances at one stage in life can be mitigated by better circumstances earlier or later in life (Graham 2002: 2008).

The life course approach has given renewed intellectual vigour to the political economy inspired materialist and neo-materialist explanations in that all three life course models direct attention to biographies of disadvantage and the cumulative effect of disadvantage on health over time. In particular, many of the studies in this field have shown that it is the cumulative effect over time of low income in combination with other indicators of poverty such as, low birth weight, poor educational attainment and poor employment conditions that accounts for inequalities in health (see Shaw *et al.* 1999, Lynch *et al.* 2001, Graham 2002).

Applications to understandings of healthcare

The principal application of the political economy perspective to understanding healthcare relates to the commodification of healthcare. Capitalist political economies have been identified as 'commodifying' health by introducing market principles into healthcare in three main ways. First, it is argued that healthcare has become dominated by technologically driven forms of curative medicine (pharmaceuticals and biotechnology), which are developed by transnational corporations primarily for private profit (Navarro 1976, 1986). Global corporations generate local demand for specialist 'curative' drugs, which puts pressure on national healthcare systems and increases inequalities in access to healthcare (McKinlay and Marceau 2002). Second, capitalist medicine is based on treating the individual consumer's health needs while obscuring from its frame of reference preventative 'up-stream' measures, which address the structural causes of ill-health. Most notably, from a Marxist perspective, the *social and economic* causes of ill-health are frequently left unaddressed. Third, capitalist medicine affects the everyday work and working conditions of health professionals. It is argued that late capitalist changes in the ownership and organization of healthcare systems are eroding the ethos of professionalism, reducing the status of doctors and transforming the nature of everyday medical work (McKinlay and Marceau 2002). One commentator has described contemporary medical work as assembly-line medicine – 'working on the factory floor with an MD degree' (Stoeckle 1987: 250). In order to illustrate the application of the political economy perspective to understandings of healthcare, we are going to focus on the latter – the changing employment conditions of healthcare workers and, in particular, the Marxist inspired theory of the proletarianization of the medical labour force.

The proletarianization of medicine: What is it?

The proletarianization of medicine thesis suggests that in advanced capitalism the autonomy of physicians is increasingly subjected to corporate and/or state regulation and control (bureaucratization), such that physicians have less control over their conditions of employment (Oppenheimer 1973, McKinlay and Arches 1985, McKinlay and Stoeckle 1988). Proletarianization involves occupations becoming more subordinate to the requirements of capitalist production. Thus, just as economic restructuring and labour market reforms have meant that other workers have lost control over the conditions of their work environment and terms of their remuneration, similar trends may be affecting doctors (Barnett et al. 1998: 196). The proletarianization thesis essentially challenges the prevailing physician dominance thesis which is well known and can be traced to the writings of Elliot Freidson (1970a, 1970b). Freidson links the professional dominance of the medical profession to the medicalization of society – the extension of medical control over more and more aspects of everyday life (see Chapter 6 for a discussion of medicalization). Freidson distinguished between medical *dominance* and medical *autonomy*. By dominance, he referred to the ability of physicians to direct and control other healthcare workers. By autonomy, he referred to the ability of physicians to exercise control over the organization and terms of its own work. Elston (1991: 61–62) has refined the concept of medical autonomy to illustrate its three primary components: *economic autonomy* refers to the right of physicians to set the terms of their remuneration, *clinical autonomy* refers to the right of physicians to determine standards of performance, assess professional competence and exact discipline procedures. Finally, *political autonomy* refers to the right of physicians to act as health experts and direct health policy. The proletarianization thesis states that physicians are being stripped of this collective form of autonomy. Advocates of the proletarianization of medicine thesis have made it clear that the challenge to physician dominance should be viewed as an incremental one and is neither universal nor unchallenged (McKinlay and Arches 1985), but that the thesis is growing in acceptance (McKinlay and Marceau 2002).

Related theories that draw attention to the declining power and autonomy of medicine are the 'de-professionalization' and 'post-professionalization' theses. De-professionalization (Freidson 1970b, 1994, Haug 1973) refers to the process whereby the clinical leadership role of physicians is weakened over time as they lose their monopoly over their unique qualities: most particularly their exclusive knowledge base, their clinical autonomy and public esteem. De-professionalization emphasizes the role of increased knowledge of health amongst the laity, or in Haug's (1973: 195) terms, 'the revolt of the client' as presenting a major challenge to medical autonomy. Post-professionalism (Kritzer 1999) refers to a loss of professional occupations' exclusivity over knowledge because of the proliferation of information technology and differences in the way that knowledge is applied through increasing specialization in the professions (Nancarrow and Borthwick 2005: 900). These theories, though related to the proletarianization thesis, focus less on the *economic conditions of employment* as the key determinant of change in medicine's autonomy. They are more clearly related to the work of the classical social theorist, Max Weber ([1922] 1978: 43–46, 339–348, 926–955) who identified the ways in which some occupations have risen to dominance by developing 'social closure', or exclusionary strategies, such as an extended formal education, in order to ensure their status and position in society.

The proletarianization of medicine: What is the evidence?

Broadly across advanced Western capitalist societies, questions about the power and autonomy of medicine have arisen in the wake of the introduction of neo-liberal healthcare cost-saving strategies and management principles (Nancarrow and Borthwick 2005). Neo-liberalism refers to the re-emergence since the 1970s of economic liberalism (a doctrine which suggests that economic development through the free market is a more desired route to economic growth and political liberty than state involvement in the shaping of economic development). Commentators have pointed to the centrality of two key features of neo-liberal economics which demonstrate the proletarianization of medicine thesis:

- The introduction of new public management in healthcare
- Re-organization of the healthcare division of labour (particularly to allow para-medical workers to take on medical tasks).

New public management in healthcare

At the heart of the new public management or *new managerialism* approach to healthcare is the introduction of private-sector business practices into state-owned healthcare systems, which is done in the name of securing better value for money, improving quality of care for a given budget and securing more accountability over what providers do (Barnett *et al.* 1998). It situates the state and service users in a neo-liberal partnership with each other with the goal of developing more cost-efficient and user-friendly/patient-centred services. The rhetoric of new managerialism is compelling, emphasizing the promotion of 'excellence of service delivery', 'quality' and 'choice' alongside discourses of 'empowerment' and 'user involvement' (see also Chapter 3). The growing popularity of this discourse in healthcare makes it difficult for any group to counter this managerial logic (Gilbert 2005). However, the success of neo-liberal (market-driven) policies in driving greater efficiencies in healthcare systems has not gone unchallenged (see, e.g., Moran 1999, Diderichsen 1995, Pollock 2004). In addition, demands associated with this neo-liberal approach for public accountability, inter-disciplinary working and responsibility for spending sit uncomfortably with traditional values of professional self-regulation, professional autonomy and professional clinical autonomy. The goal of patient-centred care emphasizes the needs of the service user over the medical profession on whom greater pressure is exerted for flexibility in working practices and in the organization of healthcare services and for the evaluation of their service provision through external performance indicators (Nancarrow and Borthwick 2005: 898). The introduction of new managerialism in healthcare systems has been enabled by new forms of medical management information systems (MMIS). MMIS can record and monitor, on behalf of the state and corporate owners of healthcare, the productivity as well as clinical outcomes of healthcare providers (such as hospitals) or individual practitioners (Barnett *et al.* 1998).

Looking at the impact of these changes on the medical profession in individual countries is also instructive. According to McKinlay and Marceau (2002: 381), in just 25 years, the US healthcare service has been historically transformed from a predominantly fee-for-service system controlled by the medical profession (fees paid directly by individuals to medical practitioners for medical services) to a corporatized system of payments to medical practitioners dominated by increasingly concentrated and globalized financial and industrial interests. As a result, where physicians should work and how much they should be paid is largely determined by others. In addition, physicians in the middle of the twentieth century tended to act as independent agents, free from administrative oversight and formal accountability (McKinlay and Marceau 2002). By contrast, in the United States today, the use of 'managed care' is widespread. Managed care refers to a system that controls spending by closely monitoring the provision of healthcare through the use of fixed payments systems, restrictions on patient care pathways and increased oversight of physicians' clinical decisions. According to Hartley (2002: 183), 'managed care is premised on maximising efficiency (i.e., containing costs) and enhancing market performance (capturing consumer market share)'. Clinical autonomy (especially, the technical content of care) has also been undermined in various ways. For example, physicians have to work to clinical practice and patient insurance company guidelines:

less individual

> ...the choice of treatment (e.g. which medication can be prescribed) is often determined by what is allowed by a patient's insurance or by the physician's employer. All clinical actions are scrutinized on a regular basis, and a deviant practice behaviour is highlighted and corrective steps taken to ensure future conformity with overall practice norms. (McKinlay and Marceau 2002: 390–391)

Finally, increased consumerism has been fostered by the state and corporate providers of healthcare through facilitating increased patient access to information on healthcare care providers (hospitals as well as individual practitioners). Through the use of the Internet, patients today can approach healthcare providers with knowledge which was once private, such as the personal and professional biography of physicians, including their education, their employment history, and the frequency and success of any legal actions taken against them (McKinlay and Marceau 2002: 399).

In the United Kingdom, the state remains the largest healthcare provider, but the state has increasingly adopted neo-liberal economic policies across the healthcare system. Although Moran (1999) has argued that the impact of changes to the United Kingdom's largely state-controlled system on the clinical autonomy of its doctors is less than physicians in the privatized healthcare system of the United States, similar trends of proletarianization of physician work are identifiable. Governments have re-structured the organization of state-owned healthcare services to include quasi-markets or 'internal markets' in the belief that they would create efficiencies, widen choice and provide greater accountability in the purchasing of health services. The development of internal markets refers to a managed market, as opposed to a free-market approach, which is based on the separation of purchaser from provider within healthcare. The main purchasers under this new arrangement are Health Authorities who shop around for the best deal for the populations they serve. National Health Service (NHS) Trusts were set up and can tender for contracts in various health authorities. What these changes have meant for physicians in the United Kingdom and elsewhere is increasing evaluation of medical interventions (Hyde *et al.* 2004). The accountability of physicians' work is promoted through the concept of 'clinical governance', which was introduced by the Labour Government in 1997 (DoH 1997) and is overseen by the National Institute of Clinical Governance (NICE) and the Commission for Health Improvement (CHI). Essentially, clinical governance demands that the standard of service to be provided by healthcare providers is set out and regularly audited. Managerial control over medical practice is most evident in the utilization of review procedures and the increasing use of protocols and guidelines for clinical activity based on the concept of 'evidence-based practice'. Commentators have pointed to the ways in which evidence-based practice may be viewed as a double-edged sword for the medical profession. On the one hand, it may act as a possible way for the medical profession to cry off the imposition of external controls by adhering to 'scientifically-proven' interventions across categories of patients. On the other hand, it may serve to undermine the clinical autonomy of individual practitioners to provide individually tailored patient-centred care and subject them to a new type of technicality (Armstrong 2002, Harrison 2002, Checkland 2004). As McKinlay and Marceau have noted,

> While originally motivated by concern over the quality of care, clinical practice guidelines are welcomed by corporatized medicine and serve to curtail extraneous and costly procedures and to streamline the production process. (2002: 390)

Nettleton *et al.*'s qualitative study of physicians' experiences of the modernization of the NHS also suggests that the use of patient protocols and evidence-based guidelines holds contradictions for practitioners in relation to the autonomy they have over their work. Guidelines and protocols were considered to be helpful when physicians were new to an area or on the margins of their specialism, but frustrating when they were not funded or not appropriate for a particular patient group. Similarly, evidence-based medicine was useful in terms of being able to efficiently answer questions but most practitioners were also critically aware of the limitations of the methodologies (randomized control trials) behind the recommendations (Nettleton *et al.* 2008: 341).

In essence, however, the increased bureaucratization of knowledge within the NHS circumscribed the day-to-day work of all of the physicians in their study.

Further evidence of the proletarianization of medicine in the United Kingdom lies in the White Paper on professional regulation: *Trust, Assurance and Safety – the Regulation of Health Professionals in the 21st Century* (DoH 2007). This outlined the government's intention to remove the right of the General Medical Council (GMC) to adjudicate on fitness to practice matters. In addition, it has been proposed that the GMC itself should be reformed such that the medical profession is no longer the majority stakeholder. The medical majority council and the right of professional self-discipline lie at the heart of professional autonomy. This further incursion into medicines' professional autonomy came on foot of a report by the Chief Medical Officer, Sir Liam Donaldson (DoH 2006a), entitled *Good Doctors, Safer Patients*. This report made recommendations for the reform of medical autonomy following the high-profile inquiry into Harold Shipman, the UK General Practitioner who was found guilty of the murder of, at least, 250 patients.

The impact of new managerialism can also be seen in recent changes in the New Zealand healthcare system and, particularly, in changes to the contracts of GPs. Dating from the development of a universal healthcare system in the 1930s, New Zealand had, like the Republic of Ireland, a dual health system with hospitals financed largely by direct allocation, and general practitioner (GP) services funded by fee-for-service subsidies and patients. As a consequence, GPs retained greater economic autonomy over their employment conditions in terms of where they could locate and in their earning capacity than hospital-based doctors. The structuring of primary care has been radically altered since the 1990s in broadly similar ways to the UK restructuring of GPs into Primary Care Trusts (PCTs). In New Zealand, Primary Health Organizations (PHOs) were introduced in 2001 to address inequalities of access to services and the lack of co-ordination between primary and secondary providers. According to Barnett and Barnett, the introduction of PHOs represents 'a fundamental shift in national primary health care policy' (2004: 61). In particular, it alters GPs contractual structures away from an individual to a population focus (although this has been emerging among primary care organizations for some time), and from a fee-for-service system to a funding approach stressing capitation with reduced co-payments (payments made by patients to the individual physician to supplement state payment) and inter-regional distribution of funds based on population need. Apart from this economic re-structuring of GP remuneration, what is also significant in terms of the proletarianization thesis is that PHOs were introduced, despite strong criticism from GPs as represented by the New Zealand Medical Association and the Independent Practitioner Association Council of New Zealand (IPAC).

Re-organization of the healthcare division of labour

We turn now to the re-organization of the healthcare division of labour as evidence for the proletarianization of medicine thesis. This is some-times referred to as the de-regulation of healthcare markets as new healthcare providers, aided by de-regulation, come to undertake some of the specialist tasks traditionally controlled by physicians. Most notably, medicine's monopoly right to prescribe and treat have been foregrounded as the hallmarks of physician professional dominance (Freidson 1970a). Therefore, the case of nurse prescribing is particularly instructive in terms of the proletarianization thesis. Legislation for nurse prescribing is currently in place in several Western countries including the United States, United Kingdom, Australia, New Zealand, Sweden (ICN 2004) and the Republic of Ireland. Specifically in the United Kingdom, nurse prescribing has now considerably advanced. Since May 2006, nurse *independent* prescribers can prescribe nearly all licensed drugs for any condition within their scope of expertise and also some controlled drugs for specific conditions (DoH 2006b). However, to date there is little evidence that nurse and other non-physician pre-scribing is having a proletarianizing effect on medicine in terms of de-skilling physicians or affecting their earning power (Britten 2001, Appel and Malcolm 2002, Mazhindu and Brownsell 2003).

Nancarrow and Borthwick (2005) explain the limitations of nurse prescribing in threatening physician dominance in terms of demarca-tion strategies between healthcare disciplines. Nurse prescribing is considered a form of vertical substitution involving the delegation of tasks 'across disciplinary boundaries where the levels of training and expertise (and generally power and money) are not equivalent between workers' (Nancarrow and Borthwick 2005: 909). As a conse-quence, the adoption of higher-order tasks by lower-status workers does not bestow on them equivalent economic or political autonomy, nor does it detract from the earning power or status of the delegating profession. Rather, it enables physicians to divert themselves from caring for groups of patients that are not very financially rewarding (Hartley 2002). Recent research confirms this description of nurse prescribing (Hales *et al.* 2007). In the case of supplementary prescribing, which is based on the joint development between doctors and nurses of a patient-care plan before prescribing by the nurse can begin, nurses reported the continuation of unequal partnerships with doctors. Collaboration took the form of nurses actually writing the care plans and doctors 'signing them off' (Hales *et al.* 2007). Thus, the case of nurse prescribing does not support the proletarianization thesis of medicine. This, therefore, leads us to a final discussion of the evidence against the proletarianization thesis.

Evidence against proletarianization: The countervailing powers thesis

According to Marxist theory, the logic of capitalism is that even the most revered professions will be enrolled into the mass of workers, alienated from control over the terms and conditions of their work and thereby reduced to proletarian status. However, as Annandale (1998: 226) has remarked it takes a great 'leap of faith' to define physicians as members of the proletariat. Or, as in the words of McKinlay and Arches (1985), how can someone earning, say $100,000 annually, be a proletarian? (cited in Barnet *et al.* 1998: 194). The countervailing powers theory seeks to theorize this scepticism over the uni-directional demise of medical dominance (Light 1993, 2000, Freidson 1994, Harrison and Politt 1994, Hafferty and Light 1995).

The countervailing powers thesis suggests that the impact of changes in healthcare delivery systems on medical dominance is not so clear cut. Some moves appear to undermine the professional powers of medicine, while others serve to enhance it (Annandale 1998: 234). In particular, the work of Hafferty and Light (1995) and Hartley (2002) suggests that countervailing pressures to medical dominance occur as a result of the complex interplay of diverse forces, interests and institutional powers (such as state policy, corporate and consumer and professional interests) creating complex changes through a system of alignments. The countervailing powers thesis can account for professional ascension as well as decline, but we are now going to focus on the ways in which the countervailing powers thesis can account for medicine's counter moves against proletarianization. Research has pointed to three principal mechanisms or countervailing pressures through which physicians resist proletarianization:

(1) *Physician Management Alignment* (the usurpation of new management logic by physicians becoming the administrators).
(2) *Physician Professional Licence* (the 'zone of discretion' at the clinical level which allows for circumvention of standardized protocols of care).
(3) *Re-stratification of medicine* (a hierarchical re-divisioning of labour within medicine which undermines the authority of some sub-groups of the profession but enhances the overall power of medicine).

Taking these in turn, it is argued that doctors can resist proletarianization by colonizing key employment positions within the new management and health policy arenas. The close involvement of doctors in health policy is what Klein (1990: 700) refers to as the 'politics of the double bed' giving doctors an advantage over other allied health professions. By infiltrating management in particular, it is argued that the new managerial logic may be diluted through the introduction of a different set of priorities that can once again bridge the medicine–management power gap. In other words, it has been argued that the growth of bureaucratization is likely to have less effect on doctor autonomy if the orders come from other doctors (Barnett *et al.* 1998: 198). However, at the level of the workplace there is both evidence supporting administrative collusion with physician interests – a *physician-administrative alignment* (Leicht *et al.* 1995, Light 2000, Hartley 2002) – and evidence to the contrary (Coburn 1993, Hunter 1994, Hafferty and Light 1995, Hartley 2002). For example, Hartley (2002) notes in her study of the context of obstetric healthcare across a number of healthcare organizations in the United States that administrative decisions, at times, uphold physician dominance and, at other times, challenge physician jurisdiction. Nonetheless, she notes that administrators in highly managed care contexts are more willing to show more overt concern with costs in their decisions surrounding hiring and use of healthcare providers. Consequently, in these healthcare contexts, administrators are more likely to challenge physician jurisdiction (e.g., in the expansion of nurse-midwifery programmes of care) when the ability to meet consumer demands is at stake. This attests to the strength of the *administrator–consumer alignment* over *a physician–administrative alignment* (Hartley 2002: 200).

The second mechanism of resistance to proletarianization is what Freidson (1994) refers to as 'a zone of discretion' or professional licence enjoyed by doctors in their everyday clinical practice. It is proposed that this professional freedom allows them to counter or resist the imposition of managerial control, as represented by the increased use of protocols and guidelines for clinical practice and review procedures. Whilst research has shown that doctors regard protocols as inhibiting their ability to exercise their clinical judgement and a threat to their autonomy (Tunis *et al.* 1994, Lawton 1998, Lawton and Parker 1999), other research in the context of nurse prescribing suggests that doctors may view protocols as a decision-making aid that can be violated at their discretion (Parker and Lawton 2000, Hales *et al.* 2007). In addition, US-based research has suggested that doctors may circumvent the imposition of widespread use of diagnostic related groups (DRGs) which, in the United States, governs the payment by treatment programme and length of stay for specific diagnosed condition by engaging in 'clinical charades' (Hafferty and McKinlay 1993) or 'perverse behaviours' such as the temporary discharge and re-admission of patients (Hunter 1991 cited in Annandale 1998: 240).

The final mechanism identified through which physicians may resist proletarianization is through *re-stratification*. Freidson (1994) suggests that the medical profession is becoming divided into an elite group of medical specialists, educationalists and higher administrators who have more authority to orchestrate control over the employment conditions and work of their junior, non-specialist colleagues. It is argued that this re-stratification allows for some proletarianizing of the work of the 'rank and file' whilst maintaining the overall power of the institution of medicine. However, the validity of the re-stratification thesis would seem to be highly dependent upon the performance of the rank and file in delivering a quality and cost-effective health service (Coburn *et al.* 1997 cited in Barnett *et al.* 1998: 198). Evidence of how governments are willing to 'step-in' with legislation designed to control the profession as a whole when matters appear to be going wrong was provided earlier in terms of the UK Government's proposed reforms to remove the right of the GMC to independently control disciplinary matters on foot of the Shipman Inquiry and the New Zealand government's re-organization of GPs into PHOs.

Conclusion and new directions for healthcare

The political economy perspective has been instrumental in highlight-ing the role of economic and class relations in shaping our health and the organization of our healthcare. In relation to understanding the application of the political economy perspective to understandings of health we may conclude the following from the above discussion. First, the theory helps us to understand how access to material resources such as an adequate income, good employment conditions and good housing, as well as neo-materialist resources such as access to an unpolluted local environment, good transport, healthcare and leisure facilities contribute towards good health. The political econ-omy theory thus broadens the dominion of healthcare policy from narrowly defined curative medicine towards more 'joined up thinking' across the domains of economic and social policy.

Second, the saliency of political economy theory can be seen in relation to other competing theories on inequalities in health. One fruitful direction in research on inequalities in health has been a com-bination of the cultural/behavioural explanation and the materialist explanation as derived from the political economy perspective. Whence combined, theories of social class inequalities in health can take on board the proposition that individuals have choices (agency) over their adoption of adverse health-risk behaviours (such as in rela-tion to smoking, exercise, diet, etc.), whilst also linking these choices to the material and cultural constraints of the social milieu in which people live. We have suggested that Bourdieu's concept of habitus is a strong theoretical route for combining these concerns. In addition, the political economy perspective has been drawn into a fruitful research debate with functionalist and psychological theories through the psychosocial explanation of inequalities in health. To date, the debate has developed in adversarial terms – in large part because of the consequences of such arguments for the direction of health policies and healthcare expenditure – but we have pointed to the ways in which psychosocial theories which focus on emotions and health are not necessarily incompatible with Marxist materialist understandings of health. They are linked – in theory – through Marx's theory of alienation. The life course approach is another way in which the saliency of the explanations derived from a political economy per-spective can be operationalized in combination with other explana-tions in multi-dimensional models. The life course approach has added further empirical weight to the political economy theory by highlighting the ways in which sustained levels of material and neo-material (individual and systemic) disadvantage adversely affect health over time. Internationally, the life course approach has been developed through longitudinal cohort data (e.g., Poulton *et al.* 2002, Osler *et al.* 2003, Batty *et al.* 2004). However, further research might develop ways to build longitudinal designs into qualitative work, not only in terms of retrospective biographical studies (e.g, Emslie *et al.* 2003, Oliffe 2008) but also in terms of prospective longitudinal quali-tative studies. Such research could add a deeper understanding of how individuals negotiate the impact of disadvantage over time, whilst also exploring the emotional as well as the material impact of disad-vantage on health.

Turning now to the contribution of the political economy perspec-tive in understanding healthcare, we have suggested that a political economy perspective seeks to critically illuminate the processes and consequences of the increased role of market forces (commodification) in the production and supply of healthcare. In this section of the chapter, we focused on the political economy inspired theory of the proletarianization of medicine and a review of the evidence for and against the impact of the proletarianization of medicine in some Western countries is summarized in Table 2.1. Although the concepts of proletarianization versus medical dominance have been a feature of this field of research for over 25 years, there are possibilities for reinvig-orated research debates on this issue. In many European countries, neo-liberal economics and corporatization of healthcare systems are only now becoming embedded in the organization of healthcare, as economically centre right governments confront the challenges of providing excellence in healthcare whilst purchasing the tools (phar-maceuticals and bio-technology) of this healthcare from global cor-porations. Also, even in our brief overview of these trends in Anglophone countries, there remain important differences in the ways in which nation states are handling the corporatization and bureaucra-tization of healthcare, as well as some differences in the ways that the medical profession is responding. Thus comparative research can help tease out broad trends as well as important differences (see, e.g., Moran's comparison of new managerialism in healthcare systems in the United States, United Kingdom and Germany (Moran 1999) and Donelan *et al.*'s (1999) comparison of citizen's views of healthcare change across five nations). The contrasting healthcare systems on the island of Ireland (North and South) could make a fascinating case study in which to compare and contrast the employment conditions

TABLE 2.1 The proletarianization of medicine: A summary

Proletarianization Theory	Evidence for	Evidence Against
The autonomy of physicians is increasingly subjected to state regulation/corporate control, such that physicians have less control over their conditions of employment, and have become, like any other employee, working for a wage	Change from fee-for-service to salaried employees and erosion of professional self-regulation of medical profession (e.g., in the US, Republic of Ireland, UK and New Zealand). Erosion of physician clinical autonomy through increased management control over the content of medical work through the utilization of review procedures and the increasing use of protocols and guidelines for clinical activity (most Western developed countries). The loss of the monopoly power of medicine over certain medical tasks and the demand for flexibility in workforces.	The medical profession remains economically powerful and retains a high degree of power over terms of remuneration. The medical profession is still professionally dominant in setting the terms of health policy and healthcare work on the ground. It has retained this position because of: (a) its ability to occupy positions within new managerial/corporate elite; (b) retain professional freedom to counter clinical governance and (c) re-stratification (medical specializations) in the profession which keeps the overall power of the profession in tact.

and levels of proletarianzation of consultant physicians working in Northern Ireland in the NHS by comparison to those in the Republic of Ireland. Traditionally, the medical profession in the Republic of Ireland has been more effective in maintaining self-regulation and setting the terms of its remuneration. However, a fundamental change has been signalled in the Medical Practitioners Bill, 2007 (DoHC 2007), which seeks to bring the regulation of physicians in line with that of the United Kingdom – for example, establishing a lay majority on the Irish Medical Council, establishing statutory requirements for the maintenance of professional competence and public hearings on disciplinary matters. Yet, despite the parallels in this proposed legislation with the UK legislation referred to above, it is likely to have a different impact in the Republic of Ireland, not least because of established higher levels of privatized healthcare in Ireland.

There is also important comparative research to be done in how the new developments, such as the case of nurse prescribing or midwifery-led care, emerge in different jurisdictions. We noted in the above discussion that increasingly national governments are de-regulating healthcare markets to allow allied health professionals to take on some core medical skills. We also concluded that currently nurse prescribing does not support the proletarianization thesis of medicine. Yet, such developments are in their infancy in many jurisdictions and, thus, so too is the proletarianization thesis in relation to these processes. Finally, there are likely to be many differences, not just at the state/national level but also in terms of how individual organizations adapt and respond to these changes as, for example, in Hartley's (2002) study of differences in levels of managed care in the United States as discussed above. Thus, the political economy approach is a useful theoretical framework for conducting comparative case studies of healthcare organizations in terms of how they adapt and respond to late capitalist restructuring of healthcare.

CHAPTER 3

Social Interaction Theory, Health and Healthcare

Introduction

The roots of social interaction theory stretch way back to the 1800s, but it was predominantly during the 1960s and 1970s that it was invoked and in turn shaped by theorists undertaking the earliest classical qualitative studies on health and healthcare. In this chapter, we explore the central principles of social interaction theory with reference to its historical development that can be traced back to the methodological ideas of Max Weber (1864–1920) and George Simmel (1858–1918). Interpretive thinking is theoretically close to the intellectual tradition of 'interactionism', or 'symbolic interactionism' developed within the Chicago School of sociology, prominent from the 1920s until the 1950s (Glaser and Strauss [1967] 1999), in spite of the two perspectives having emerged from entirely separate sources (Outhwaite 2005). Given their theoretical proximity, we will explore these two conjointly in the first section on the principles of social interaction theory.

We then go on to examine the application of social interaction theory to our understanding of both health and healthcare. These sections are awash with classical works, but here we also consider more contemporary empirical research that draws on this perspective. In the conclusion, we consider social interaction theory with reference to future directions for health research in the context of recent developments in social theory more widely.

Principles of social interaction theory

Social interaction theory, often referred to as *interpretivism* or simply *social action theory*, refers to a broad theoretical perspective that emphasizes the significance and centrality of subjective[1] meanings associated with social actions and institutions. While there are many diverse perspectives under the broad umbrella of social action theory (as indicated in Table 3.1), a central thread throughout is an understanding of society as socially produced through the micro-interactions that occur between individuals in everyday life. In this sense, human beings are believed to themselves create or develop the rules and normative practices within their culture, rather than merely responding to the dictates of social structure. Since interpretivists broadly view humans as active in shaping their world, this has implications for how they view social change. Because individuals are considered to be active knowers, change is possible from the bottom-up rather than being imposed from above. Interpretivism is fundamentally about understanding social processes by beginning from the inside, at the level of the world of individuals, rather than in attempting to explain social processes from the outside (Outhwaite 2005). Thus, in a crude sense, interpretivists are less concerned with explaining social processes through social structure, that is, through the influence of large-scale institutions on people's lives, but rather are concerned with people's subjective meanings, with social action and interaction, and with individual agency. Therefore, the appropriate level of analysis for interpretive, or humanistic, theorists is the individual. However, the extent to which the various theoretical perspectives under the general banner of social action theory challenge the notion of social structure acting on individual behaviour tends to vary.

Let us reel back to the work of Weber to get a sense of the genesis of contemporary social interaction theory. In contrast to positivist sociological positions purporting that reality is 'out there' waiting to be discovered, Weber ([1947] 2002: 178) instead held that 'the acting individual attaches a subjective meaning to his [sic] behaviour – be it overt or covert, omission or acquiescence'. Thus, for Weber, social action is invested with meaning, with the individual taking into account the

---

[1] While acknowledging a degree of definitional variation about the meaning of 'subjective' within social theory, the concept is widely used to refer to a social actor's perceptions, experiences and interpretations of the world and the micro-dimension of the social realm. This is in contrast to the concept 'objective' that refers to the macro-component of the social that is deemed (by some theorists) to heavily determine social action. The macro-dimension is concerned with social structure and how society imposes order on and constrains social actors.

TABLE 3.1 Social interaction theory (interpretative or humanist theory)

Verstehen	Phenomenology	Symbolic interactionism	Ethno-methodology	The social construction of reality
Max Weber (1864–1920) Georg Simmel (1858–1918)	Alfred Schutz (1899–1959) Edmund Husserl (1859–1938) Martin Heidegger (1889–1976)	Herbert Blumer (1900–1987) Erving Goffman (1922–1982)	Harold Garfinkel (1917–)	Peter Berger (1929–) Thomas Luckmann (1927–)
A social action is underpinned by an individual purpose that is orientated in its course by the expected conduct of others, Social action theory emphasizes the need to understand values and meanings of action.	Objectivism and the notion of meaning independent of the mind or being is rejected.	People's actions are based on the symbolic meaning they assign to things and these meanings arise from social interaction. People interpret their own and others' actions and actively construct their social world.	People continually classify both their own and other people's statements and actions through processes and methods; social actors themselves 'make' social order.	Social reality extends beyond the immediate; however, it is humanly produced and does not acquire an ontological status apart from the human activity that produced it.

behaviour of others, and in turn being influenced by this; behind a social action – one of its causes – is the individual's purpose or intention brought about by taking cognizance of the expected behaviour or conduct of others. In *Economy and Society* (Weber [1922] 1978), Weber delineated four types of social action, namely instrumentally rational action (motivated by a goal); value-rational action (motivated by a value); affectual action (motivated by affect or emotion) and traditional action (motivated by traditional practices). The sociologist's ability to *understand* social phenomena was central to Weber's work and he used the German word *verstehen*, meaning 'understanding', in his historical research to refer to the endeavour of the social scientist to comprehend both the intention of human action and its context.

Georg Simmel, a German and a contemporary of Weber, was originally a positivist, but shifted position in the course of his writings (Ørnstru 2000). Although Simmel ([1908] 1959) distinguished between various levels of social reality from the microscopic psychological dimensions of social life to the more macro-components of the social and cultural changes occurring in the contemporary period of his life, interaction was central to his understanding of society and the world (Ritzer and Goodman 2003). Simmel held that interactions were driven by human needs, instincts and goals, and were not random or aimless (Ørnstru 2000). To cope with the complex nexus of events, actions and so forth, which he referred to as the *content* of social life, human beings imposed order in the form of patterns, or *forms* on everyday events (Ritzer and Goodman 2003). Although it has been noted that aspects of Simmel's work exhibit realist tendencies in which society is treated as a material structure (Coser 1965 cited in Ritzer and Goodman, 2003), Simmel's later work is strongly interpretivist, affording him a central place as one of the first interpretivist thinkers.

Social interaction theory: Phenomenology

Interpretivism also encompasses phenomenology, a perspective within which objectivism and the notion of meaning independent of the mind or being is rejected (McNamara 2005). Phenomenology is associated with social theory through the work of Alfred Schutz. Although phenomenological ideas can be linked back to the philosophers of ancient times (Heidegger [1927] 1982), phenomenological thinking was advanced in the late nineteenth and early twentieth centuries by Edmund Husserl ([1913] 1982) and his student Martin Heidegger

([1927] 1982). Husserl's phenomenology, referred to as descriptive phenomenology (Lopez and Willis 2004) encompasses an approach to knowledge whereupon our *experience* of things is sought by bracketing out concerns about whether such things actually exist or not (Outhwaite 2005). In this sense, experience becomes the only source of knowledge, 'the real subject matter, as well as the ultimate arbiter, of philosophical truth' (Ferguson 2001: 233).

Heidegger, a student of Husserl, developed a separate branch of phenomenology referred to as interpretative or hermeneutic phenomenology. It differs from Husserlian phenomenology in that it is concerned with exposing what is normally hidden in human experience. Thus, it is not concerned with describing core concepts and essences of phenomena, but extends to looking for meanings in everyday life events (Lopez and Willis 2004). Such meaning is not always transparent to the person experiencing the phenomenon but may be accessed through the experiences that he or she narrates. Thus, it is what individuals experience rather than what they consciously know that is the basis of investigation (Lopez and Willis 2004).

Through developing the concepts of Husserl, Schutz initiated phenomenological sociology in the 1930s (Outhwaite 2005). Husserl's concept of 'lifeworld' was used by Schutz to refer to the everyday common-sense social world, prior to theoretical interpretations by social scientists. Schutz noted that humans make sense of their world through a 'stock of knowledge' that has become taken-for-granted (Outhwaite 2005: 113), and which provides humans with reference systems on which to base interpretations (Harste and Mortensen 2000). He also held that meaning was constructed from the outset in the social world, rather than being 'some inner subjective state' (Harste and Mortensen 2000: 180). Schutz ([1967] 2002: 32) distinguishes between 'my lived experiences of you' as distinct from '*your* subjective experiences'. Schutz expanded on the components of interpreting the actions of others in the social world, and distinguished two aspects of this interpretation, namely the objective and the subjective:

> Objective meaning is the meaning of the sign as such, the kernel, so to speak; whereas subjective meaning is the fringe or aura emanating from the subjective context in the mind of the sign-user [...] The subjective meaning that the interpreter *does* grasp is at best an approximation to the sign-users intended meaning, but never that meaning itself, for one's knowledge of another person's perspective is always necessarily limited. (Schutz [1967] 2002: 34, 37)

Social interaction theory: Symbolic interactionism

As indicated, social interaction theories encompass the tradition of symbolic interactionism, a term devised by the Chicago sociologist Herbert Blumer (1900–1987) in 1937 (Outhwaite 2005). Blumer's work was influenced by the writings of George Herbert Mead (1863–1931) on how the self develops through interaction with others. Blumer was adamant that the social world should be studied in its natural form ('naturalistic inquiry'), rather than in abstraction.

> [...] such direct examination permits the scholar to meet all the basic requirements of an empirical science: to confront an empirical world that is available for observation and analysis; to raise abstract problems with regard to that world; to gather necessary data through careful and disciplined examination of that world; to unearth relations between categories of such data; to formulate propositions with regard to such relations; to weave such propositions into a theoretical scheme; and to test the problems, the data, the relations, the propositions, and the theory by renewed examination of the empirical world. (Blumer 2002: 67)

Blumer identified four key premises in symbolic interactionism. The first of these was that people, both individually and collectively, were 'prepared to act on the basis of the meaning and the objects that comprise their world' (Blumer 2002: 68). The second related to the notion that people's association with one another occurs through a process of 'making indications to one another and interpreting each others indications'. The third premise is that both social and collective acts 'are constructed through a process in which the actors note, interpret, and assess the situations confronting them'; and finally, the fourth point relates to the dynamic nature of the social world – that 'the complex interlinkages of acts that comprise organization, institutions, division of labour, and networks of interdependency are moving and not static affairs'. Blumer highlighted the methodological implications of these central conceptions, insofar as an understanding of the actions of individuals can occur only when the researcher sees objects in the social world as those being studied see them.

Interactionism became a competing perspective to structural functionalism (see Chapter 1), the former espousing theories as sensitizing concepts with a tolerance for informality and plurality, and the latter advocating theoretical precision, systematization and generalizability

(Outhwaite 2005). In later years, interactionist thinking was developed further in the United States through the work of Erving Goffman (1922–1982) and Harold Garfinkel (1917–present).

Goffman's first book, *The Presentation of Self in Everyday Life*, published in 1956, detailed the manner in which humans are constantly engaged in performances and 'interaction rituals'. In keeping with social interaction theories, Goffman's work focuses on face-to-face interactions; social life is likened to a theatre. Goffman (1969: 14) defines face-to-face interaction as 'the reciprocal influence of individuals upon one another's actions when in one another's immediate physical presence'. Goffman constructs the activity of a particular participant on a given occasion as a *performance*; others involved in the situation are considered to be either observers or co-participants. What Goffman refers to as a *part* or *routine* is the 'pre-established pattern of action which is unfolded during a performance and which may be presented or played through on other occasions [...]' (Goffman 1969: 14). The performance has two components, the *front* and the *backstage*. The front is the part of the individual's performance that operates to define the situation for the observers. In addition, when the individual presents himself or herself, the performance will tend to project society's accredited values, more than does the person's behaviour overall.

The backstage is the place where 'the impression fostered by the performance is knowingly contradicted' as a matter of course' (Goffman 1969: 97). In the backstage, the front can be dispensed with, and it is here that 'illusions and impressions are openly constructed' (Goffman 1969: 97). According to Goffman (1969: 202–204), tact is employed when, 'the audience and outsiders act in a protective way in order to help the performers to save their own show', and '[...] at moments of crisis for the performers, the whole audience may come into tacit collusion with them in order to help them out'. Goffman's notion of 'performance' has been the subject of criticism, in so far as it suggested that individuals were constantly acting in public encounters, and did not allow for negative cases or resistance to social codes of conduct (for an overview of critiques of Goffman's idea of 'performance', see Manning (1992: 51–55)). The earlier construction of 'performance' as occurring in all social interactions was modified by Goffman himself in his later work where the notion of performance was acknowledged as being limited in its applicability (Manning 1992). In the third section of this chapter on the application of social interaction theory to understandings of healthcare, we will consider Goffman's work on asylums and his notion of total institution.

Social interaction theory: Ethnomethodology

Garfinkel, a contemporary of Goffman, was concerned with how social order was maintained in micro-level encounters, and developed the branch of interpretivism called 'ethnomethodology'. Ethnomethodology refers to the investigation of 'expressions and other practical actions as contingent ongoing accomplishments of organized artful practices of everyday life' (Garfinkel 1967: 11). Ethnomethodology is concerned with how people continuously classify both their own and other people's statements and actions through processes and methods (Harste and Mortensen 2000). Garfinkel drew attention to the implicit and implied meaning in everyday social interaction. However, he indicated that it is impossible to make completely explicit the body of common-sense knowledge exchanged within a group; indeed when he requested of his students an exhaustive and literal report of a specific interaction, they were unable to produce it (Harste and Mortensen 2000).

In ethnomethodology, the notion that social order is 'out there' as a 'reality' that people internalize through social norms is rejected (Poloma 1979: 193). That said, Garfinkel did view 'social facts' as central to sociological phenomenon, but these 'social facts' were the outcome of the methodological activities of members, and 'locally, endogenously produced' (Garfinkel 1991: 11) rather than determined by social structures beyond individuals. Within ethnomethodology, it is proposed that social actors themselves *make* social order (Poloma 1979). At the same time, ethnomethodology is not just about the micro-level of social interaction, but is also concerned with the artful mechanisms people use to produce what for them can be either large-scale or small-scale structures (Ritzer and Goodman 2003). As Ritzer and Goodman (2003: 375) note, '[...] ethnomethodologists are interested in *neither* micro structures *nor* macro structures; they are concerned with the artful practices that produce *both* types of structures'.

Social interaction theory: The social construction of reality

Another influential interpretive sociologist is Peter Berger, a student of Schutz. Along with Thomas Luckmann, Berger co-authored a major volume, *The Social Construction of Reality* (1966), in which the theoretical perspectives on society presented in Berger's earlier text *Invitation to Sociology: A Humanist Perspective* (1963) were developed. Unlike eth-nomethodology that holds that the social world exists contemporane-ously to those experiencing it, Berger believed that social reality extends beyond the immediate, in other words, that there is an objec-tive social reality acting back in a structuralist type of way (Poloma 1979). Berger and Luckmann explain this as follows:

An institutional world [...] is experienced as an objective reality. It has a history that antedates the individual's birth, and is not accessi-ble to his [sic] biographical recollection. It was there before he was born, and will be there after his death. This history itself, as the tradi-tion of the existing institutions, has the character of objectivity [...] The institutions, as historical and objective facticities, confront the individual as undeniable facts. The institutions are *there* [emphasis in original], external to him, persistent in their reality, whether he likes it or not. He cannot wish them away. They resist his attempts to change or evade them. They have coercive power over him, both in themselves, by the sheer force of their facticity, and through the con-trol mechanisms that are usually attached to the most important of them. (Berger and Luckmann [1966] 2002: 46)

For Berger and Luckmann ([1966] 2002: 46), however, this objective reality was 'a humanly produced, constructed objectivity', brought about through a process of 'objectivation'. As Berger and Luckmann ([1966] 2002: 46) clarify, '[...] despite the objectivity that marks the social world in human experience, it does not thereby acquire an onto-logical status apart from the human activity that produced it'. Thus Berger and Luckmann's perspective contests that social reality is a social fact in its own right, but rather consider it to be socially pro-duced and communicated through human interaction. This is distinct from the perspective of Durkheim ([1895] 1982: 50) who identified 'social facts' as possessing 'the remarkable property of existing *outside* [our emphasis] the consciousness of the individual'. While interpreta-tive theories tend to focus more heavily on human agency than on the constraining effects of social structure, Berger and Luckmann's perspec-tive might be interpreted as theoretically close to structuration theory (Giddens 1976, Archer 1988, 1990, Parker 2000), where much is made of the notion that '[...] man [sic] (not of course, in isolation but in his collectivities) and his social world interact with each other. The prod-uct acts back upon the producer (Berger and Luckmann [1966] 2002: 46).' However, interactionists have been accused of a one-sided concentration on individual motivation and action as an explanation for social life, just as structural functionalist (Chapter 1) theorists have been regarded as only taking the influence of social structures into account (Bhaskar 1989a). The trick, according to these critics, is to adopt a social theory that can take due account of both. We might think back here to the quotation from Marx in Chapter 2, where he stated,

> Men [sic] make their own history, but they do not make it just as they please, they do not make it under circumstances chosen by themselves, but under circumstances directly found, given and transmitted from the past. (Marx [1852] 1954: 10)

The influence of social interaction theory on research methodologies

Before moving on to consider how social interaction theories have been used in attempting to explain health and illness, we need to clarify briefly the relationship between such theoretical notions and methodology.[2] Since social action theories take as their starting point human interaction, methodologies that are influenced by interpretative approaches generally use qualitative analytical techniques. These involve the investigation of a phenomenon in depth, using small sample sizes relative to quantitative studies. In addition, since qualitative methodologies tend to proceed initially in an inductive manner, that is, by building interpretations from an engagement with data, it is unlikely that a researcher would approach such a study with one particular interaction theory in mind with a view to testing its applicability. Qualitative researchers are generally not in the business of entering the research field already armed with a theory to test – that

---

[2] 'Methodology' is a contested concept, with some accounts viewing it as a research model, including the methods and overall framework employed, in practice lending itself to as many methodologies as studies, since each study roll-out has its own individual process (Sarantakos 1998). Sarantakos (1998) also notes that methodology has also been perceived in a more overarching sense as encompassing the research principles of a particular paradigm such as qualitative or quantitative, so that one may speak of qualitative or quantitative methodologies. There are a number of ways of conceptualizing methodologies between these two (Sarantakos 1998). Methodology encompasses questions about how knowledge may be acquired (Porter 1996) and the philosophical principles mediating the research process.

is the realm of quantitative work. This is not to say that the findings of such a qualitative study would not support the theoretical propositions of one or other interpretative theory. Nor is it to suggest that qualitative research proceeds in an 'anything goes' type of fashion, of which it is often accused (sometimes with justification). Rather, we are simply cautioning that when it comes to the execution of a research study, say for example in the health sphere, it is relatively rare to find any of the theoretical approaches hitherto outlined followed to the letter in explaining the raw data gathered. Rather, the spirit of interpretive social inquiry mediates the process.

A number of qualitative methodological approaches have been influenced by social action theories, and the methodological stance adopted in a specific piece of health research tends to be fairly explicit in most published papers. However, the extent to which the methodological procedures have been strictly employed is often nebulous because of the very limited space afforded to methodological considerations in published research articles.

Applications of social interaction theory to understanding health

In this section, we consider the application of social interaction theory to understanding health in relation to a number of themes as follows:

- The social construction of health and illness
- Interpretative studies of stigma
- The application of grounded theory in health studies
- The social construction of mental disorders
- Lay experiences of health and illness
- The interpretative influence on the sociology of emotions
- Phenomenology and nursing research.

The social construction of health and illness

Since social interaction theories are primarily concerned with how individuals create society in their everyday interactions, health and illness are believed to be socially constructed rather than physiological facts. To put this another way, what 'health' or indeed 'illness' means is not standard and unchanging across all social groups, nor across historical periods. Rather people – both lay and professional – through the patterns and practices of their culture, are active in shaping what counts as health and what counts as illness. As Radley (1994) notes, just what it means to say that someone is ill is not clear-cut, but rather depends upon those evaluating the situation. There may be discrepancies between a medical judgement of a set of symptoms (and even what actually gets labelled as a symptom) and an individual's assessment of his or her bodily experiences of symptoms. This discrepancy has been used to explain why apparently a considerable number of people in the community have clinical pathologies (according to dominant biomedical definitions) for which they do not seek medical help, while others with very minor symptoms apparently do (Dunnell and Cartwright 1972, Cartwright and Anderson 1981, Scambler *et al.* 1981). Interpretivists would argue that this arises because people have mechanisms, constructed through social interaction, for evaluating what constitutes symptoms of ill-health and for making decisions about whether or not to seek medical help.

An interpretative perspective would also hold that medical judgements likewise are not objective, impartial assessments by 'disinterested' scientists, because medical knowledge is similarly produced and modified by human beings acting within the context of their culture. Of course medical scientists undertake experiments in laboratories and produce apparently 'objective' results, but constructionists would argue that what areas to research, how to conduct an experiment, what generalizability means, what counts as 'statistically significant' evidence and so forth are all concepts mediated by social and cultural contexts and are far from watertight and infallible. Moreover, there are good reasons, predominantly relating to vested interests, that raise questions about how objective medical scientific results really are. For example, in a study of 811 scientific papers in leading medical and molecular biology journals, Krimsky *et al.* (1999) found that over a third of the primary authors located at research institutions in Massachusetts had a considerable financial interest in their own studies. In addition, it has been found that where drug studies have been funded by the manufacturers, the researchers are more inclined to arrive at a more positive conclusion regarding the drug's safety, efficacy or cost-effectiveness compared with the situation where the research has been funded by a non-profit organization (Krimsky 2001). What this suggests is that human actions are influencing the results of studies dealing with diagnosis and treatment of diseases rather than some impartial set of principles developed in the scientific world. In this sense 'scientific' results are the construction of human conduct and are manipulated and shaped according to human interests.

Given that humans seem to have some kind of culturally influenced mechanism for interpreting their own symptoms, and that scientists have been charged with creating research conclusions to suit themselves, both 'lay' people and 'experts' can be said to decide the meanings of health and illness and its management from within their social contexts. What makes this perspective interpretative is that the starting point of analyses is the micro-level of the social actors, who are considered to be active in shaping society.

Interpretative studies of stigma

As indicated earlier, influenced by the perspective of symbolic interactionism, Goffman (1963) analysed how people present themselves to others in the course of social interactions. One aspect of some interactions was the manner in which stigma was managed. In *Stigma: Notes on the Management of Spoiled Identity*, Goffman (1963: 14) distinguishes between stigmatized persons that are 'discredited' and 'discreditable'. In the case of the former, the stigmatized person assumes that his or her differentness is immediately perceptible, and therefore the management of tension in social encounters is central, whereas in the second category, the person's stigma is neither known to the observer nor perceivable by him or her, and the management of information is central. Stigmatized people more generally incorporate standards from wider society, to a greater or lesser extent, and are aware of the degree to which they deviate from them (Goffman 1963). Goffman (1963: 45) has noted a socialization process whereby 'the stigmatized person learns and incorporates the stand-point of the normal, acquiring thereby the identity beliefs of the wider society and a general idea of what it would be like to possess a particular stigma'. In the case of inborn stigma (as might be the case with a congenital physical handicap), individuals might have been protected from freely expressed disapproval through information control from early in life.

Goffman's analysis of stigma has been used since in a number of later studies in explaining patients' experiences of mental illness (Hall *et al.* 1993, Herman 1993) and physical illness and disability (O'Farrell 2002, Lee and Craft 2002). Scambler (2004) notes that our understanding of stigma has not shifted much since Goffman's work, and sets about re-framing our interpretation of stigma. He revisited the concept of stigma by a reappraisal of his own *hidden distress model* developed to understand stigma related to epilepsy (Scambler 1989). Scambler's critique of his own earlier model highlights many of the criticisms of social interactionist theory, with its overbearing focus on institutional order and symbolic frameworks and its failure to sufficiently problematize social structures and sites of power. In his re-framing, Scambler elucidates the weaknesses of his earlier analysis in accepting biomedical definitions of epilepsy, in presupposing epilepsy to be a personal tragedy and in suggesting that those with epilepsy passively accepted others' responses to their condition. Thus, while descriptions of social action theory often draw attention to the agency this perspective affords to the individual in actively shaping his or her world, as we highlighted earlier in this chapter, empirical studies such as Scambler's – by his own later assessment – paid less attention to the subject as an active agent of social change in challenging the social structure, focusing instead on the biographical impact of having a particular chronic condition. As Scambler (2004: 36) himself put it, both himself and early American labelling theorists 'failed to invigorate their interactionism with conflict theory, thus leaving power out of the equation'. Scambler (2001b, 2002, 2004) advocates, as a corrective to this shortcoming, the inclusion of analyses of the role of the economy and state mediated by money and power respectively in understanding how stigma is created.

The application of grounded theory in health studies

To return to the earlier period – the 1960s – before the shifts that have marked recent decades of sociological theorizing, Barney Glaser and Anselm Strauss developed a qualitative methodological strategy referred to as grounded theory. Although grounded theory is often associated with symbolic interactionism, Glaser and Strauss acknowledge criticisms of the Chicago tradition as 'a less than rigorous methodology, and an unintegrated presentation of theory' ([1967] 1999: vii). In fact, both theorists came from different philosophical traditions. Strauss studied at the Chicago school and was influenced by interactionism, while Glaser had come through the Department of Sociology at Columbia University associated with Robert Merton's quantitative methodological stance. Between them, they created a methodological strategy for generating theory from data based on clear systematic procedures in terms of coding data and testing hypotheses that arise during the research process.

The interactionist tradition is manifest in many aspects of the strategy, particularly in terms of the importance of grounding theory in 'everyday reality' as well as the notion of people actively shaping their worlds (Strauss and Corbin 1990: 23–25). This methodological strategy was used by its progenitors to study dying, and has since also been use in many studies to describe and explain the experience of illness. For example, Dingley and Roux (2003) used a grounded theory strategy to investigate the experience of inner strength among older Hispanic women with chronic illness, while Ackerson (2003) invoked the central techniques of grounded theory to study the experience of parenthood from the perspective of people with a severe mental illness.

The social construction of mental disorders

Scheff's (1974) work on the labelling theory of mental illness is a classic example of how social action theory is brought to bear in explaining mental illness. Scheff analysed how the medical model plays a part in creating a deviant condition, and how patient characteristics rather than objective sets of symptoms mediate the process of diagnosis. The label itself, Scheff noted, is related to a change in the person's self-concept and behaviour. Thus, deviance is deemed to arise in the dynamics of interaction during which people apply meanings to specific kinds of behaviours. In defending his theoretical perspective against positivist critics, Scheff (1974: 444) draws on Blumer's (1954) notion that concepts and theories may have a sensitizing rationale that is separate from their 'literal truth value'.

Rosenhan's (1973) classic study where empirical evidence is drawn from the actual experiences of people is a good example of how people get labelled with a mental diagnosis, in other words, with how psychiatric disorders are socially produced. In this sense, it may be located in the domain of the social interaction theory. Rosenhan describes an 'experiment' in which eight people from a variety of social backgrounds were admitted to a psychiatric institution, after fabricating symptoms of psychosis. Each claimed to have heard voices that said three words, 'empty', 'hollow' and 'thud'. Apart from these contrived symptoms, these pseudopatients behaved in their normal way once admitted. Nonetheless, all but one were admitted with a diagnosis of schizophrenia, and all were afforded the label of schizophrenia 'in remission' on discharge.

Rosenhan's paper brings out strongly the way in which meanings get created in human interaction and through prior understandings. For example, hospital staff wrote up in case notes aspects of one pseudopatient's (genuine) life history to make his situation consistent with contemporary accounts of schizophrenia. In other words, conventional traits of schizophrenia were 'read into' aspects of this person's everyday behaviour. Similarly, with the other pseudopatients everyday behaviours were redefined as symptoms of a psychiatric pathology. For example, their writing up of field notes as part of the research was interpreted as an aspect of their psychiatric pathology in nursing records. What Rosenhan tried to demonstrate was that the diagnosis of schizophrenia is not objective, absolute and irrefutable, but rather negotiated, produced and socially derived. While Rosenhan was not explicit about which specific theoretical perspective, if any, mediated his work, this social constructionist perspective beginning with the experiences of the human subject tends to place him within an interpretive position.

Two further issues are of note here regarding Rosenhan's analysis. One concerns how the agency of human actors is presented in the study, and the other the way in which social structure is theorized. With regard to individual agency, what Rosenhan exposes more than anything else is the relative helplessness of the ordinary individual in contesting diagnostic labels: '[h]aving once been labelled schizophrenic, there is nothing the pseudopatient can do to overcome the tag' (Rosenhan 1973: 253). As noted in relation to Scambler's (1989, 2004) analysis of stigma, referred to earlier, this seems at variance with the agency usually afforded within social interaction theory to human beings, who are supposed to be actively shaping their world. It indicates that the ideals of theoretical perspectives can throw up diverse interpretations in actual empirical studies. Rosenhan's study instead seems to indicate that while the actions of individuals create broader patterns in society, these act back on individuals, allowing some social actors (such as medical and nursing staff in this instance) greater leeway to be creative compared to others. He also noted, however, that the perceptions and behaviour of staff 'were controlled by the situation, rather than being motivated by a malicious disposition' (Rosenhan 1973: 257), bringing us to the issue of the existence and impact of social structure. Rosenhan was clear that there was a reality beyond that immediately created in the course of interaction, arguing that '[a] psychiatric label has a life and an influence of its own' (Rosenhan 1973: 253). Similarly, Rosenhan theorizes power and powerlessness from a structural perspective while interspersing this with actual examples from both his own and others' experiences as pseudopatients.

Lay experiences of health and illness

If we move from the 1960s and 1970s to the 1980s, we see a proliferation of studies on lay experiences of health and illness. In a shift in emphasis from more structuralist approaches such as Parsons' sick role (see Chapter 1) and overarching concepts like medical dominance, studies of lay experiences of health and illness take as a starting point social interactions at the micro-level and attempt to explain how people construct, experience and explain illness from their perspective. In this sense, the philosophies underpinning social interaction theory mediate many of these studies. Some of the most influential studies on lay perspectives published in the journal *Sociology of Health and Illness* during the 1980s have been identified by Julie Lawton (2003) as Bury's (1982) paper on 'biographical disruption', Charmaz's (1983) article on 'loss of self' and William's (1984) work on 'narrative reconstruction'.

'Biographical disruption' refers to the manner in which the experience of chronic illness can prompt a major revision in thinking of a person's self-concept and biography (Bury 1982). Located within a symbolic interactionist perspective (Lawton 2003), 'loss of self' refers to the way in which people with extreme disability experienced their former self-image degenerate without the reconstruction of an equivalent alternative one (Charmaz 1983). 'Narrative reconstruction', the third central concept identified by Lawton, concerns the way in which those with long-term chronic illness make sense of their illness by bringing together components of their previous experiences and biography with aspects of the present (Williams 1984). As Williams notes,

> Narrative reconstruction is an attempt to reconstitute and repair ruptures between body, self and world by linking-up and interpreting different aspects of biography in order to realign present and past and self with society. (Williams 1984: 197)

Williams (1984: 177) developed the concept to address 'how and why people come to see their illness as originating in a certain way', and traces the influences of this particular stance back to a range of studies on lay beliefs or folk theories. While Williams acknowledges that the notion of narrative cannot be traced directly to any specific school or tradition, his sense of biography is associated with Peter Berger's work, and 'narrative' is seen as the 'cognitive correlate' of biography. For Williams ([1984]: 178), narrative is 'a process of continuous accounting whereby the mundane incidents and events of daily life are given some kind of plausible order', giving his work a distinct flavour of social interaction theory.

The interpretative influence on the sociology of emotions

In these 1980s studies that focus on the social construction of illness, we begin to see a shift in emphasis to situating the body as a focus of analysis, extending social action theory into a newer theoretical category of the sociology of the body. Through the analyses of symbolic interactionists in the last few decades, an interest in the sociology of emotions has also opened up (James and Gabe 1996, Bendelow and Williams 1998, Sandstrom *et al.* 2001), a realm hitherto deemed to be that of psychologists. Invoking an interactionist perspective, Hochschild (1983) draws attention to the social aspect of emotions and the manner in which they can operate as signals between the self and the environment. She argues that the social dimension of emotions comes into play during social interactions in how we conduct and express ourselves. Freund (1990) proposes that a useful approach for studying distressful feelings, society and health may be facilitated through an emphasis on the emotionally expressive, embodied subject, who is active in the context of power and social control.

We also see the application of social action theory, and more specifically phenomenology, in Bendelow's (1993) advancement of the sociology of emotions in relation to the role of gender in the construction of pain perceptions. Her analysis points to gender differences in the impact of emotions on the perceptions of pain, with women far more likely to link the two in response to direct questions; indeed men were frequently reluctant to ascribe the status 'pain' to emotional types of suffering. Nonetheless, when men opened up in the interview situation, they were able to discuss feelings of vulnerability in relation to emotional pain. Several male participants believed that expressing pain would label them as 'sissy' or effeminate. What Bendelow's analysis points to is that meanings and definitions of pain for both sexes incorporated feelings, emotions and indeed spiritual and existential components, challenging the conventional scientific wisdom that pain amounts to physical sensations. In addition, Bendelow noted that feelings of punishment and self-blame mediate the experience of pain, and these may contribute to the self-identity of the sufferer.

While Bendelow's analysis elucidates the manner in which individuals actively construct their pain definitions, she does link these to structural aspects of gender. For example, in relation to the finding that participants believed that women were 'naturally' better at coping with pain than men, Bendelow (1993: 289) associates this to women's historical connection with the domestic sphere where bodily functions are foregrounded compared to the public world of '"higher" cultural and mental processes' more heavily occupied by men. Bendelow (1993: 291) thus links the subjective experience of pain to the 'perceived "objective" reality of the world and other people'. It should be noted that Bendelow writes of a *perceived* objective reality, which is in keeping with a phenomenological perspective which purports that there is no objective reality outside of human knowledge or consciousness.

Phenomenology and nursing research

Phenomenology has also been invoked in nursing research in attempting to explore how lay people experience or make sense of illness. An example is Beck's (1992) study of women's experiences of post-natal depression that invokes a descriptive phenomenological approach. In keeping with Husserlian descriptive phenomenology, Beck assumed that there was an essential structure of post-natal depression, and that this could be specified and separated out from its context. From the detailed narrative accounts of 7 women, Beck identified 11 cluster themes that described the core essence of post-natal depression as they were consciously experienced by participants, without reference to the context.

Much phenomenological research in nursing focuses on the lived experience of participants, an area of research that has come under considerable criticism in recent years for its misunderstanding of both Husserl and Heidegger. Phenomenological nursing research has in particular been the subject of criticism by Crotty (1996, 1998), Paley (1997, 1998) and McNamara (2005). The controversy is related to the manner in which nursing research is deemed to have amalgamated other research traditions such as humanistic psychology and American intellectual thinking associated with symbolic interactionism (Crotty 1996). As McNamara (2005: 697) observes, 'Nursing phenomenology fails to get behind the mundane and banal which throw a veil over the objects of pre-reflexive experience.' Phenomenological enquiry ought to be about 'a contemplation of the objective inherent in the subjective and unearths the *what* buried in the *how* and *why* of their experiences' [emphasis in original] (McNamara 2005: 703). He and others argue that nursing phenomenology is erroneously concerned with subjective experiences and meanings imparted within a culture rather than setting these aside and getting back to the things themselves. It might be noted that while nursing phenomenology claims to associate with philosophical phenomenology, with its aim to uncover the things themselves, what researchers in this field are really doing is more like the sociological approach advocated by Schutz, where the object of analysis is the common-sense stock of knowledge that people use to guide their interpretations and actions.

Applications of social interaction theory to understandings of healthcare

Social interaction theory explains healthcare by beginning at the level of social interaction to achieve a greater understanding of the social organization of healthcare. According to this perspective, what we experience as healthcare is not a social fact in the sense that it acts upon us in a deterministic way, but rather is constructed within everyday social interaction. The perspective has given way to various accounts of the social organization of healthcare such as 'total institution' and 'negotiated order' (that we explain further on), and to analyses of relations within the health sector between various groups such as lay people and professionals, and professionals themselves. What this broad church of ideas share is a focus on how reality is constructed at the micro-level, although the relationship between the micro- and the macro-levels (agency and structure) is variously interpreted. In this section, we consider applications of social interaction theory to understandings of healthcare in relation to the following themes:

- The social organization of healthcare
- Lay and professional relationships in healthcare
- The occupational socialization of health workers.

The social organization of healthcare

Goffman, whose work was influenced by the tradition of symbolic interactionism, as indicated earlier, produced an account of how mental
health services are socially organized. Goffman drew on empirical examples of interaction (and sometimes the control of interaction) (primarily
from the fieldwork of others) between patients and staff in mental hospitals to construct the notion of 'total institution'. Total institution refers
to an umbrella of shared (though not perfectly delineated) characteristics, a central one of which is the control of the activities of sleep, play
and work in the same location and controlled by the same single authority (Goffman [1961] 1998: 101). Residents in such institutions are subjected to 'batch' treatment in that they are treated in the same way and
have to engage in the same activity together. Goffman used the concept
of total institution to explain the round of life in a mental hospital.

Strauss (the US interactionist referred to earlier) *et al.* ([1963] 1998:
249) use the term 'negotiated order' to refer to the 'complicated process
of negotiation, of bargaining, of give-and-take' that occurs when hospital staff disagree over matters relating to patients. They refer to dis-
agreements about, for example, the best place to locate a patient, and
her clinical status (e.g., what 'getting better' means) (Strauss *et al.*
[1963] 1998: 249). The concept of negotiated order encompasses an
understanding of social order as something that is not static or pre-
given, but rather as dynamic and continually reconstituted. However, a
criticism directed at this perspective is that it understates the constraining potential of social structure (see Allen 1997). However, Allen identifies a more guarded theorization of the scope of negotiation in Strauss's
later work in which he concedes that 'not everything is either equally
negotiable or – at any given time or period of time – negotiable at all'
(Strauss 1978: 252 cited in Allen 1997: 500).

The concept 'negotiated order' was also taken up to explain interactions between nurses and doctors in healthcare settings. The first of
these interaction studies, against which many of the later studies were
compared, was Leonard Stein's (1967) analysis of a telephone conversation between a nurse and a doctor in a US context in which an interaction style called the 'doctor-nurse game' was first identified. Stein
described this as follows:

> The cardinal rule of the game is that open disagreement between
> the players must be avoided at all costs. Thus, the nurse can com-
> municate her recommendations without appearing to be making a

recommendation statement. The physician, in requesting a recommendation from a nurse, must do so without appearing to be asking for it. (Stein 1967: 699)

Thus, to maintain the normative hierarchical relations between the nurse and the doctor, the nurse was required to hide her knowledge, skills and information and adopt a deferential disposition. Several later studies contested that the doctor–nurse game represented the dominant pattern of interaction between doctors and nurses, particularly where nurses were interacting with junior doctors (Hughes 1988, Porter 1991, Walby and Greenwell 1994), and even Stein and his colleagues acknowledged that power relations had shifted when they revisited the doctor–nurse game two decades later (Stein *et al.* 1990).

Svensson (1996: 381) used the notion of negotiated order to explore how nurses' power and function has altered because of revisions in the 'negotiation context' in recent years, namely, the widening terrain of chronic illness that requires greater nursing input, as well as organizational reforms that have facilitated a new context for co-operation between doctors and nurses. What we see in the case of Svensson's (1996) findings is empirical support for a theoretical proposition, that of 'negotiated order', developed from an interpretivist tradition.

However, in a study in Britain involving similar empirical work, Davina Allen (1997) found little empirical support for the notion of negotiated order in inter-occupational relations between nurses and doctors. While, in the course of research interviews, nurses and doctors indicated uncertainty and discordance about their shifting role demarcations, observations at the clinical site found that 'nursing, medical and support staff carried out their work activities with minimal inter-occupational negotiation and little explicit conflict (Allen 1997: 505)'. Thus, while qualitative researchers do not usually enter the health research field armed with theories to test, what we see emerging in research findings into healthcare settings is support for specific theoretical propositions in certain social locations, and a challenge to such propositions in others, even where both pieces of research are coming from the same broad theoretical tradition such as interpretivism.

Lay and professional relationships in healthcare

If we move on to a somewhat different component of healthcare, namely relations between professionals and lay people, there is no shortage of studies that invoke interpretivist thinking in order to illuminate aspects of how healthcare is executed. For example, influenced by the tradition of ethnomethodology, du Pré (2002) conducted a study of the micro-interactions between a doctor and patients to investigate the nature of communication between the two parties. Drawing on Mishler's (1984) distinction between the 'voice of the lifeworld' (the social and personal contexts of everyday life) and the 'voice of medicine' (the biomedical and technical perspective), du Pré focused on the issue of how 'lifeworld' (everyday) talk relative to 'medical' talk was managed in the course of the encounter. Her analysis pointed to the notion that biopsychosocial communication could be achieved in a relatively short space of time, invoking a variety of communication techniques. This type of interaction was found to be particularly favoured by patients when their self-image or social status were under threat.

Similarly, Lehtinen (2005) used a methodological strategy based on ethnomethodological conversation analysis to study the manner in which doctors check out a patient's understanding of information imparted during genetic counselling. Drawing on 10 video-recorded sessions in a genetics clinic in Finland, Lehtinen (2005: 595) notes that what occurred in the clinical context reflected the orientation towards 'the benign order of everyday life' (Maynard 2003) insofar as good news or positive information was overt and emphasized, while bad news or negative news was cloaked and played down.

A further example of the way in which social interaction theory is used to explain the patient's perspectives on the delivery of the health services comes from McCoy's (2005) study of the doctor–patient relationship in the case of those with HIV. McCoy used 'institutional ethnography' as a methodological strategy that involved focus group interviews to gain insights into social relations, particularly institutional work processes and associated modes of knowledge that shape the doctor–patient relationship. The author focused in particular on how participants constructed the notion of 'good doctoring'. Rather than concentrating solely on an individual participant's attitudes or beliefs, data were analysed with an emphasis on the interface between the individual and institutional work processes. McCoy found that socially marginalized participants had positive regard for the notion of doctors being respectful during the consultation. The minimizing of social distance and not acting aloof or superior on the part of doctors were also positively received, as was the doctor accepting the client's different (and in some cases, unstable) way of living. For those clients whose lives were affected by poverty, addiction, mental illness or illegal activities, good doctoring was also characterized by the doctor extending his or her care beyond that expected in typical cases.

Finally, doctors' facilitating an understanding of information, and not merely imparting it, was constructed by participants as good medical practice.

Doctor–doctor relations have also been the subject of study by interpretivists. Paul Atkinson's (1995: ix) analysis of the 'everyday work and talk of haematologists' concerns how haematologists 'produce and reproduce knowledge about particular medical conditions' and how they seek to have this knowledge justified and legitimated. Atkinson sought to highlight the 'work' involved in the social construction of medical knowledge. Atkinson (1995: ix) deliberately excluded direct interactions with patients from his analysis in order to draw attention to the manner in which patients 'are constructed and reconstructed as objects of a medical discourse that is enacted away from the patients themselves'. Atkinson notes how much of sociology of health and illness is limited to the cultural construction of illness, that is, the notion that people's response to a disease or disorder is socially constructed and subject to cultural variation. What Atkinson (1995) draws attention to, however, is that the apparently common body of knowledge shared among doctors, and upon which they make diagnoses based on analysing signs (manifestations that may be perceived – seen, heard or felt by an observer) and symptoms is also culturally derived.

The occupational socialization of health workers

Social interaction theory has also informed studies that attempt to illuminate aspects of the occupational socialization of health workers who deliver healthcare. Becker *et al.*'s (1961) ethnography of medical students at the University of Kansas detailed the socialization of doctors as they progressed through medical school. The study revealed details of the students' routines, their attempts to be strategic about what was required in tests and exercises, covert aspects of their culture, the manner in which they acquired medical values and their negotiation of life in a hospital or clinic. Ethnographic studies of medical education have also been conducted in Britain. Atkinson's (1997) Scottish study explored the transmission of medical or surgical knowledge in the course of clinical learning. Sinclair (1997) focused on the culture of medical education and found that students learned to co-operate with one another in passing examinations and in covering up for one another in relation to aspects of clinical work. Sinclair also considered how the status acquired by medical students relative to other students amalgamated with other factors and lent itself to feeling of exclusivity. Studies on the socialization of nurses have also invoked the tradition of interpretivism. Drawing on grounded theory, Melia's (1987) study of the occupational socialization of nurses highlighted the discrepancy between the idealized version of nursing presented in colleges of nursing and the reality of daily nursing practice.

Conclusion and new directions for healthcare

We have indicated in this chapter that social interaction theories have in common an interest in analysing the routine interactions of everyday life, and are concerned with unpacking these in order to understand the social world. Nonetheless, in spite of their shared interest in taking interaction as a starting point in explaining how society works, as we have seen, social interaction approaches exhibit considerable variation. The multiple strands tend to differ in the interpretation of the concept of social structure, for example, in terms of whether or not it is bestowed with an objective reality and how much or how little it is seen to impact upon human behaviour.

In terms of their utility for better understanding health issues, social interaction theories are most useful in those areas associated with understanding the experiences of illness, illness behaviour, and how health and illness are constructed. Studies underpinned by social interaction theory often offer a depth and richness that tends to be absent from macro-sociological analyses. Arguably, this detailed analysis of the realm of health and illness enables healthcare practitioners to get greater insights into the world of illness, and closer to the bone in term of human suffering, with possibilities for facilitating a greater sense of empathy with those suffering. In addition, where the organization of healthcare is the focus of study, social interaction theories expose patterns and power relations in healthcare. In particular, studies invoking social interaction theories are especially useful in giving a voice to those in marginalized groups in society, whose own perspectives are rarely elicited. Micro-sociological studies can also be a useful means for assessing health policies insofar as people's own perspectives may be compared with how such perspectives are represented or managed at a more macro-policy level, or indeed how the impact of health policy is played out at the micro-level.

Interaction theories have been criticized for analysing interaction predominantly in a modern Western context (Harste and Mortensen 2000).

In addition, other theoretical avenues have opened up, such as feminist perspectives (see Chapter 5) and poststructuralism (see Chapter 4), that emphasize resistance to rules of social conduct, exposing some of the shortcomings of social interaction theory. Furthermore, social action theory has also been accused of having an excessive focus on immediate action to the detriment of macro-social analyses (see Scambler 2004 and Dixon-Woods *et al.* 2006) and theory development (Harste and Mortensen 2000).

While the perspectives associated with social action theory are necessarily qualitative, the recent focus on evidence-based practice in healthcare research spells a return to a heavy emphasis on quantitative methodologies and a general sense that components of reality can be identified, measured and evaluated. Problematizing aspects of social life as fluid, ephemeral, socially produced and, to some extent, elusive is often a source of frustration and irritation of those who want neat and clear research results.

In relation to ethical issues, while social action theories have the potential to enhance ethical practices in healthcare by, for example, including the perspectives of marginal groups, such theories are not without their ethical problems. As indicated, social action theories of one kind or another permeate most qualitative research, yet many of the skills associated with the most popular data-gathering technique in qualitative research, the depth interview, may present ethical challenges. It is well established in the research literature that a well-designed interview guide begins with less-sensitive issues to reduce tension, with more problematic topics held over until later (see Brannen 1988). It may well be argued that that using such tactical measures to access the richest of data is unethical insofar as respondents are lured into divulging as much as possible, perhaps more than they intended.

In terms of new directions for research, where health and healthcare studies use social action theory, we are likely to see a greater integration of the principles of social action theory with other theoretical persuasions in an effort to address the deficits of the former. This type of theoretical synthesis is evident in recent health research such as Dixon-Woods *et al.*'s (2006) account of why women consent to surgery that they do not want, whereupon an interactionist approach is combined with a Bourdieusian analysis. (For an account of Bourdieu's theory of social capital, see Chapter 1, and of his concept of 'habitus', Chapter 2.) The whole notion of looking at reality as something constructed in social interactions rather than 'out there' waiting to be discovered with a prior existence has spilled over to a whole variety of perspectives that tend to be considered as separate theoretical genres. These include feminist theory and poststructuralism; how each of these perspectives is brought to bear in scholarship on healthcare to be explored separately in this book.

CHAPTER 4

Poststructuralism, Health and Healthcare

Introduction

In this chapter we outline poststructuralist social theory as it is applied to the sociology of health and illness. There is a wide diversity of writing associated with a poststructuralist position and definitions vary depending on whether the focus is on philosophy, social science, feminism or literary studies. Indeed, poststructuralism is often defined as an intellectual movement rather than a discreet body of theory, which rejects what is popularly referred to as 'grand theory' (totalizing theories of society based on universal concepts) (see Chapter 2). Those writing within the canon of poststructuralism challenge the notion of universal and objectively founded truth claims and, generally, emphasize that all knowledge is socially constructed and historically specific. In this respect, poststructuralists often focus their analysis of society on how knowledge is constructed, not to dispute or otherwise claims to 'truth' but to reveal the social processes behind the way society is organized.

We focus on the work of the French philosopher Michel Foucault and how his ideas have been interpreted and developed in theoretical and empirical studies in the sociology of health and healthcare. This is not an easy task because as Armstrong (1997: 15) in a review of the influence of Foucault's ideas on the sociology of health and illness notes, there are '...many different readings and many different Foucaults'. What marks Foucault as a poststructuralist thinker, particularly in his later work, is his understanding that human subjectivity (the property of being a subject) is socially constructed. What he means by this is that human behaviour is socially determined. While the prefix 'post' might suggest a radical break with structuralism, here we see a much stronger line of continuity.

However, Foucault rejects Marx's notion of an underlying universal structure determining the course of human history (see Chapter 2 on Marx's concept of the mode of production) as well as the idea that social analysis can objectively define the truth of such structures (Layder 1994). He also rejects the structuralist-functionalist notion that human behaviour is governed by a set of general rules (see Chapter 1). Foucault is, instead, interested in the everyday social practices that govern human behaviour. This idea will be teased out when we unpack the theoretical principles in some of Foucault's major works.

In the first section of this chapter, we focus on a number of Foucault's works that trace the rise of modern forms of power and how these are linked to the way that human behaviour is governed and, in turn, to the way that we think about ourselves as subjects. We explain Foucault's sociological theory of the relationship between power and knowledge through a number of key concepts including the 'clinical gaze', 'disciplinary power', 'biopower', 'technologies of self' and 'governmentality'; and, finally we look at how Foucault has reworked the concept of power which goes against the grain of traditional sociological questions, such as who holds power and to what end? In the second part of the chapter, the research that we draw on develops Foucault's concepts of 'disciplinary power', 'biopower' and 'governmentality' to trace the changes that are occurring between the relations of knowledge, power and expertise that govern health and how these, in turn, produce new modes of subjectivity in terms of how we understand and act upon the self in the name of health. Finally, we consider the application of these concepts to explain shifts in the way that health is governed, particularly in the area of public health and health promotion, and through various forms of clinical governance; and how these changes impact on the relations between patient and health professional, and between that of health professionals and the state.

Foucault and the principles of poststructuralism

Foucault's analysis of modern society involves tracing the way that knowledge is linked to power in terms of how it both assumes and achieves its authority as a truth claim. In Foucault's theoretical formulation, knowledge is always implicated in relations of power because it defines the norms by which subjects come to understand themselves.

Power circulates through the discourses (specialist languages and their specific systems of meaning), techniques (strategies for targeting those who are the objects of knowledge) and practices (routine ways in which knowledge is put into effect) generated by knowledge. Power is made effective when we subject ourselves to the meanings and norms of behaviour generated by knowledge. These ideas are found in Foucault's 'genealogical' histories (those histories that trace the relationship between knowledge and power),[1] *Discipline and Punish* and *The History of Sexuality*, which we go on to discuss. Foucault accords a special status to medicine both as a dominant discourse in generating ideas about the body, health and disease and, at a much deeper level, rendering control over the vitality of the body, of life itself and the formation of self (subjectivity) as political objects of government. In Foucault's second major work, *The Birth of the Clinic* ([1973] 1976), he argues that health supplanted salvation as the quintessential modern ethic of living when modern medicine displaced the authority of religion. In his later work, Foucault (1980) argues that in the modern period, specifically from the eighteenth century onwards, social life became organized around maximizing physical well-being and health. This explains why medicine became bound up with the objectives of government.

The clinical gaze

The concept most commonly cited from *The Birth of the Clinic* is that of the clinical or medical 'gaze'. For Foucault, the clinical gaze marked a decisive break in the history of medicine. Under the auspices of public health in the later eighteenth century, the clinical gaze penetrated the social space and Foucault associates the medicalization of society with the 'positive' function that medicine would play in instilling a generalized medical consciousness about the role of health and good living:

> Medicine must no longer be confined to a body of techniques for curing ills and of the knowledge that they require; it will also embrace a

---

[1] Foucault's genealogical method differs from conventional approaches to history, which ordinarily charts a linear line of progress from the original source of ideas in the past to present day practices. The genealogical method is as Nettleton (1994: 77) describes 'a history of the present', which seeks to understand how particular ideas and practices become established as truth claims and ways of being within their own temporal framework.

knowledge of *healthy man*, that is, a study of *non-sick man* and a definition of the *model man*. In the ordering of human existence it assumes a normative posture, which authorizes it not only to distribute advice as to healthy life, but also to dictate the standards for physical and moral relations of the individual and of the society in which he lives. (Foucault [1973] 1976: 34)

In the nineteenth century the medical gaze was institutionalized in the birth of the hospital clinic where patients could be observed and examined, cases recorded and compared, treatments complied with and monitored. While medicine acquired its knowledge by observing and categorizing diseases according to the similarities and differences in symptoms, clinical anatomy based on the dissection of corpses deepened the perceptual field of medicine beyond the surface of the body and the reporting of symptoms. In death, the organic basis of disease was revealed and in this sense, Foucault argues that death no longer symbolized the limits of medical knowledge but the very possibility of its truth as a science of the human condition. As we will go on to discuss, medicine plays a formative role in what Foucault understands as uniquely modern forms of power.

Disciplinary power

In *Discipline and Punish* (1979), Foucault conceives of a new form of power that is distinct to the modern period, which he calls 'disciplinary power'. Disciplinary power refers to those techniques derived from knowledge of human behaviour for controlling, regulating and managing bodies – in other words, a form of power that is bound up with the production of knowledge and operationalized through the mechanism of surveillance. In the seventeenth and eighteenth centuries the function of disciplinary power was negative or repressive. By the nineteenth century, however, disciplinary power was expected to perform the more positive function of maximizing the utility of individuals in relation to their capacity to be productive and healthy. This power was meant to be a more efficient and lighter form of social control. In this work, Foucault argues that the human sciences (including medicine, psychiatry, psychology, penology and sociology) gave rise to new objects of knowledge, which greatly expanded the scope of surveillance. Disciplinary power makes itself felt as a normalizing force, in that it both defines what is 'normal' and encourages individuals to adhere to the normality it defines. It operates through the surveillance of individuals across multiple sites such as the school, factory, clinic and prison – those sites where individuals can be trained in disciplinary regimes that effect the correct moral disposition towards the body and the self. Discipline invokes a normalizing judgement against which individual behaviour can be judged and corrected: the observation of individuals is meticulously recorded and classified and, from such individual records, a body of knowledge about whole populations is developed. The following and much-cited quote demonstrates how knowledge is implicated in and central to the exercise of power:

> There is no power relation without a correlative constitution of a field of knowledge, nor any knowledge that does not presuppose and constitute at the same time power relations. (Foucault 1979: 27)

For Foucault, the technologies of domination implied in disciplinary power are not experienced as repressive but are rationalized in the name of social progress and are effective because they do not weigh too heavily on its subjects. In other words, we tend to accept what experts define as normal and strive to meet those standards.

Biopower

Foucault associates disciplinary mechanisms of power with a new and distinct form of administrative power from the eighteenth century. This theme is continued in *The History of Sexuality* (published in three volumes). In the first volume (1984a), he uses the term 'biopower' to capture the sense in which life itself and the vitality of the body (individually and collectively) became the political object of modern government. He conceives of biopower as operating between two poles. 'Biopolitics' is the pole of biopower concerned with the regulation of populations in terms of the specific goals of government through, for example, demographic and epidemiological knowledge and public health programmes allowing for the surveillance of whole populations. The other end of the continuum of biopower is premised on what Foucault refers to as the 'anatomo-politics of the human body'. This concerns the discipline of the individual body, for example the clinical examination measures individuals against the norms of health. The emergence of 'population' as an economic and political problem is described by Foucault (1984a: 25) as 'one of the great innovations in the techniques of power'. He shows how the governance of sexual conduct was at the heart of the problem of population and, therefore, subject to a proliferation of regulatory discourses that define the norms of sexual behaviour. Here Foucault is also concerned to understand how the moral prohibitions surrounding sexuality incited a search for knowledge about oneself and an obligation to reveal the truth about oneself – to render one's thoughts and action open to judgement.

Technologies of the self

In his later work, Foucault's emphasis on technologies of the self seeks to explain how the individual participates in the regulatory imperative of modern life by engaging in monitoring her own behaviour (Hutton 1988). A decisive point of departure from *Discipline and Punish* is his contention that the regulation of sexuality depends more on technologies of the self than technologies of power. Technologies of power refer to those discourses and practices that objectify the subject in order to control the individual for particular ends or domination. Technologies of self are those techniques or practices that we apply to our own bodies, thoughts and behaviour – in other words, how an individual acts upon herself in order to attain what Foucault (1988: 18) describes as 'a certain state of happiness, purity, wisdom, perfection, or immortality'. In short, he argues that social control is not just a matter of what other people tell us to do, but involves what we ourselves think we should do.

Foucault traces the philosophical foundations of technologies of self to ancient antiquity, when the principle of an ethical relation to self or the 'care of self' was a key organizing rule for social and personal conduct, and to Christian asceticism (which involved renunciation of earthly pleasures) where care of the self no longer referred to the good citizen and the 'art of living' but to an obligation to attend to the soul for the purpose of salvation. The Christian confession is a technique of self that entails not only the obligation to tell the truth (disclosure of the self), but to judge such truths and submit them to institutional authority. Foucault argues that from the eighteenth century this technique was adopted by the human sciences (such as medicine and psychiatry, and later psychoanalysis) not as a technique for renouncing the self but of constituting a new self – a disciplined conception of the self, which is decisively modern. The new disciplines then are part of the social and cultural forces that shape the self: scientific knowledge is enmeshed in practical reasoning through the provision of techniques for individuals to engage with self-analysis and to assert power over their own behaviour. For Foucault, the self as subject is constituted by the discourses that seek to understand it: in other words, the self has no objective status outside of those discourses and knowledge theories.

Governmentality

The emergence of the modern state from the eighteenth century saw the development of a specific set of techniques of government based on a new political rationality for integrating the individual into the utility of the state (Foucault 1988). Foucault is less interested in ideologies of the state than in the practices involved in this new form of rationality, which he called 'governmentality' (Foucault 1991). This new form of political rationality associated with the emergence of the administrative state was concerned with all aspects of human life and social relations including health, disease, morality and productivity. Foucault (1988) explains that the project of sustaining life and maximizing its vitality (whether targeting individual bodies or whole populations) is not simply considered a consequence of good government, but a condition and technique of government. The human and social sciences emerged as part of this new political rationality and became part of its political technology – the modern subject and the problem of populations became objects of science, and this knowledge became a tool of government and the basis of practical reason in the organization of everyday life. Foucault's (1988) idea of governmentality refers to a specific form of modern regulatory power or a rationality of government, which conjoins 'technologies of power' (e.g., technologies of surveillance associated with disciplinary power) and 'technologies of self' (self-regulatory practices). Governmentality does not simply refer to the power of the state to regulate (centralized power) but to a nexus of agents, disciplines (professional bodies of knowledge and their institutional settings) and technologies (techniques and strategies) that target and render measurable aspects of individual and population health and well-being.

Governmentality as a specific form of modern power is premised on knowledge as a regulatory mechanism, on the one hand, and the production of self-regulating subjects that draw on various forms of expertise, on the other. While the state remains a powerful player in the politics of regulation, governmentality is premised on the principle of 'governing at a distance' through intermediary agencies (Gordon 1991) that, in turn, are also subject to various forms of surveillance (Flynn 2002). Thus, the web of governmentality is a lot wider than the power exercised by what we think of as 'the government'. In this respect, governmentality refers to government through expertise (Rose [1989] 1999). As we will go on to discuss, Foucault's concept of governmentality has proved particularly fruitful as a theoretical framework in explaining the shift from welfare to neo-liberal policies and in raising critical questions about how we come to view the self in relation to health, and the implications this policy shift has for healthcare. Central to Foucault's concept of governmentality is his understanding of the fragmentary nature of modern society where power is no longer centralized (e.g., with the state) but diffused as an omnipresent force throughout society. Furthermore, the concept of governmentality attempts to bring together two aspects of Foucault's work, namely his emphasis on power as domination (in *Discipline and Punish*) and his concern with technologies of self and the active way in which subjects constitute themselves in the later volumes of *The History of Sexuality*. However, the apparent contradictions in Foucault's work on power are not resolved by the concept of governmentality. We now turn our attention to Foucault's treatment of power before considering how his ideas have been developed in the social study of health and healthcare.

A theory of power

In the first volume of *The Will to Knowledge: The History of Sexuality* (1984a), Foucault argues that power is *not held* by particular social groups; instead power is better understood as a force that is *exercised* in the name of social programmes to improve public health, increase productivity, expand education and so on. The utility of this kind of power is that it is diffused throughout society across multiple sites and serves multiple and complex social functions. This kind of power is most effective when it does not need to resort to the exercise of sanctions or negative power in order to shore up the sovereign power of the state. In 'Truth and Power' (1984b), Foucault describes power as 'productive' in the sense that it produces knowledge of the subject and regimes of truth in the form of discourses, techniques and practices by which subjects come to understand themselves. He specifies that the function of power is not only repressive nor its effects only negative. In describing the productive expression of how power operates, he states,

> What makes power hold good, what makes it accepted, is simply the fact that it doesn't only weigh on us as a force that says no, but that it traverses and produces things, it induces pleasure, forms of knowledge, produces discourse. It needs to be considered as a productive network which runs through the whole social body, much more than as a negative instance whose function is repression. (Foucault 1984b: 61)

The following points summarize Foucault's theory of power:

- Power is not the property of individuals, social groups (such as a dominant social class or institution) or the state.
- Power is not held but exercised, and it is exercised not from a centre point (e.g., the state) but through a myriad of power relations that are networked in a capillary-like fashion throughout society.
- Power serves multiple social functions and its effects are not uniform.
- Power, nonetheless, is all encompassing: while power relations shift, power is a force field from which we cannot escape or transcend.
- Power is not simply repressive, either in the functions that it performs or its effects: instead, power is productive in terms of its practical effects in producing new objects of knowledge, new discourses, new practices and new modes of subjectivities.

Notwithstanding the different emphases placed by Foucault over time, his work contains the common thread of the omnipresence of power. As he puts it in the first volume of *The History of Sexuality*, 'Power is everywhere...because it comes from everywhere' (1984a: 93). This position has been subject to considerable criticism because, as Eagleton (1991) observes, for a term to have any meaning, it must be possible to specify what would count as something other than it. If power is found in all interactions it becomes impossible to differentiate between different instances of the application of power (Porter 1996b). Thus, critics such as Sahlins (1993) argue that Foucault is falling into the same sort of error that compromised structural functionalists, as outlined in Chapter 1. Rather than using 'social solidarity' as the catch-all explanation for all kinds of human behaviour, Foucault is accused of substituting the equally universal notion of power. In this sense, Foucault's framework can be frustratingly ambiguous about the institutional and structural basis of how power is exercised and the effects of power (Layder 1994), which can lead to different and contradictory interpretations in the application of this theory to research.

Applications to understandings of health

In this section we explore how Foucault's ideas have been developed to explain how the ideal of the 'healthy self' takes the form it does as a contemporary mode of subjectivity. The health surveillance research emphasizes how this ideal is mobilized as a governmental strategy that targets lifestyle-related behaviours. This strategy is promoted as something more than a risk-reducing activity but as a means of actualizing the liberal goal of personal autonomy. As we are increasingly defined and invited to see ourselves as autonomous agents in relation to our own health, new tensions arise between political governance concerned with social regulation, on the one hand, and those practices that cultivate a greater sense of personal responsibility and autonomy with respect to health, on the other hand. We consider how Foucault's ideas are brought to bear in understanding how health surveillance is increasingly linked to the 'self-responsibilization' of health (Osborne 1997) under the following themes:

- The imperative of health and how the idea that we are each responsible for our own health takes hold through cultural, political and health discourses;
- The individualization of health;
- Risk surveillance and self-governance.

The imperative of health

We live in an age where health as a value is ubiquitous: discourses of health abound from threats to public health to nutritional advice, and more and more aspects of our daily living are directed towards the achievement of health. Health is increasingly commodified in the form of marketable lifestyles that cultivate an expanding market for expertise on how to live happy, risk-free and fulfilling lives that underscore a neo-liberal value system based on consumer choice, personal autonomy and self-mastery. Sociologists refer to this social phenomenon concerning the widening scope and definition of health as the 'imperative of health' or 'healthism' (Lupton 1995). Those writing within a Foucauldian theoretical framework link health promotion as a political technology constituting the active patient to the wider political rationalities of government. Health promotion has become a key strategy in the governance of health, and health promotional discourse constitutes the 'active patient' as the individual consumer who takes responsibility for her own health and well-being. The active patient signifies a discernable shift in the governance of health away from the idea that the state has the sole responsibility in protecting health to an emphasis on individual responsibility (Higgs 1989). This contrasts with the Parsonian notion of the passive patient discussed in relation to the sick role in Chapter 1.

Health promotional discourse is linked across multiple sites from the clinic to community development initiatives on healthy living, from public health promotional initiatives to the gym, and from 'healthy eating' campaigns in schools to workplace fitness and health programmes. Hence, Petersen (1997: 197) describes the scope of health promotion as 'a multi-organizational network of surveillance and regulation'. Health promotional discourse is also aligned with and finds expression through other discourses including, for example, the philosophy of 'holism' in complementary and alternative health discourses, the language of 'empowerment' by self-help groups, as well as in the expanded role of health professionals in identifying and preventing health risks through a more comprehensive approach to the patient's family history and social context. Health promotional discourse is also allied to more general cultural shifts, including the influence of an individualistic, consumerist culture and the proliferation of what Rose ([1989] 1999: xii) defines as the contemporary 'therapeutic culture of the self', where the self is defined as an individualized project of lifestyle, self-improvement and self-investment. Yet another important aspect of the cultural shifts in which health promotional discourse has become more prominent is the emergence of what the sociologist Ulrich Beck calls the 'risk society'. Beck's *Risk Society* (1992) is a seminal work in the field of 'risk studies', which is increasingly characterized by a competing variety of theoretical conceptualizations of risk (Adam *et al.* 2000, Taylor-Gooby and Zinn 2006). Beck associates the rising consciousness about risk with the transition from traditional to 'reflexive modernity'. The certainties that we once assumed lay in scientific, technological and economic progress have been undermined by a new set of conditions, including the individualization of lifestyles and the loss of social solidarity embedded in the welfare model, which promised a more equitable distribution of resources and social protection, along with a proliferation of competing knowledge claims and a plurality of value systems. Hence, while individuals have more options than ever before there is an abiding sense that the world that we live is increasingly outside of our control. The widespread apprehension that this has created has made us more reflexive about the negative global impact of scientific and technological progress, for example, the environmental risks associated with technological and industrial policy or the lifestyle risks associated with consumer capitalism. Beck argues that the kind of risks that we are faced with today are not bounded by national, social or cultural contexts (e.g., Bovine Spongiform Encephalopathy (BSE) or Creuzfeldt Jakob Disease (CJD), HIV/AIDS, Avian Flu and Severe Acute Respiratory Syndrome (SARS)); they have a global impact and are difficult to calculate and, therefore, they are often subject to competing knowledge claims. Climate change or nuclear power are good examples that illustrate these characteristics of modern risks. Today's risks are also characterized by the threat that they pose for our cultural meaning systems and social institutions: here we need to go no further than the debates about genetic engineering. As Lupton (1995) notes, in public health discourse and surveillance strategies, risk is technically defined as a measure of the probability of disease and its statistical distribution within and between population groups. Risk is further categorized as either environmental and, therefore, external to the individual or lifestyle related and, hence, assumed to be within the control of the individual (Lupton 1995).

The individualization of health

Over the last two decades, Western health policies, following the World Health Organization's health agenda, have targeted diseases associated with lifestyles, such as cardiovascular disease, cancer and diabetes and, increasingly, obesity. The policy mantra of self-care emphasizing self-management and self-knowledge is premised on the notion that the risks associated with ill-health are calculable and, therefore, avoidable through personal choices and lifestyles. This has generally entailed a shift from a focus on the structural and societal to the individual and individual psychology of behaviour. However, while it is generally observed that experts disagree about risks and how they are measured or prevented, the individualization of risk underscores the ideal of the modern subject as an autonomous individual who is free to make the right choices. For some theorists working with Foucault's concept of governmentality, how we are expected to behave in relation to health risks is premised less on prescription than on the principle that we have the capacity to be self-managing, self-regulating subjects. The ideal of the 'enterprising, autonomous self', Nettleton (1997: 220) points out, is not simply an ideological construct of the New Right, but a mode of subjectivity that is fashioned out of the techniques and practices associated with the governance of health and a 'neo-liberal governmental rationality'. What do we mean by a neo-liberal governmental rationality? While governmentality is premised on self-conduct defined in terms of the exercise of free will, its current neo-liberal form emphasizes self-governance as a way of life or a moral code of conduct, which produces a particular form of subjectivity that we can refer to as the 'entrepreneurial individual' (Petersen 1997: 194, see also Rose [1989] 1999). A central paradox noted by Petersen (1997) is that the proliferation of discourses about health risks has effectively served to privatize and, hence, individualize health in a way that not only shifts responsibility to the individual but also greatly expands the scope of surveillance.

Risk surveillance and self-governance

Risk surveillance is a key aspect of the biopolitics of health and in the shift from welfarism to neo-liberalism, governmentality studies stress how practices of governing increasingly emphasize the ideal of the active subject. This echoes Foucault's notion of technologies of the self, whereby it is not simply a matter of the welfare state being responsible for our well-being, but is a matter of our own self-regulation. This, in turn, broadens the target and scope of health surveillance. For example, in the wake of the public health crisis posed by AIDS, Zibbel (2004) traces how the new public health policy on harm reduction transformed drug users from passive clients subject to expert interventions to expert patients and consumers. Reducing the risk of HIV required a new strategy of actively recruiting drug users into services and, therefore, the target of surveillance was expanded to bring all intravenous drug users into contact with services irrespective of whether they perceived their drug use as a problem in need of treatment or not. The expertise and role of the drug professional was also expanded from drug addiction treatment to that of 'harm reduction education', the purpose of which was to 'implant in drug users the aspiration to *actively* pursue harm reduction techniques' (Zibbel 2004: 58, original emphasis). In order for this to work, drug users need to be inculcated into the new rationale and, therefore, they are encouraged to view harm reduction techniques as a question of personal choice, which are practised in the name of protecting their own health. This captures the essence of Foucault's theory of governmentality where governed subjects come to view themselves as acting or self-governing subjects.

While risk awareness is a public health strategy and health promotion is activated as a technology for encouraging the active engagement of individuals in the management of their own health, we may well argue that this can have the reverse effect in at least some areas of health prevention, perhaps best demonstrated by the case of childhood immunization. Public health interventions that target population risk, such as childhood immunization programmes, have traditionally been seen as obligatory of the 'good citizen' (Brownlie and Howson 2006), and participation has been seen as a measure of collective solidarity and public investment in good government. Following the public controversy surrounding the triple vaccine for mumps, measles and rubella immunization (MMR),[2] the rate of childhood immunization began to decline. Rather than identifying with the science of population risk, significant numbers of parents began to individualize risk in relation to the particularities of their own children's social and medical circumstances. The central paradox here is that in collectively resisting government public policy, parents were able to draw on the policy rhetoric of individualized healthcare (Hobson-West 2007) and in terms of individual resistance, they drew on the language of health consumerism

---

[2] This controversy emerged following the publication of a report in the *Lancet* of a study by Wakefield *et al.* (1998), which claimed a link between MMR, autism and inflammatory bowel disease. This has been the subject of considerable media attention and has since been strongly disputed by the medical scientific community (see in particular Patja *et al.* 2000).

(Poltorak *et al.* 2005). The case of parental resistance is revisited in the following section in the context of the implications that it raises for health professionals and the governance of healthcare.

Applications to understandings of healthcare

The extent to which health is achievable as a social objective and, perhaps more to the point, the extent to which this is achievable at the lowest cost politically and economically depends on the active engagement of individuals in their own health. Therefore, the idea of responsibility for one's own health also has implications for healthcare (Osborne 1997). In the shift from welfarism to neo-liberalism, health promotional discourse has become more central to healthcare policy where the emphasis is clearly on the active patient as a consumer and autonomous agent who makes rationale choices about appropriate practices of prevention. In the shift from passive patient to active consumer, the relationship between patient and health professional also changes (also discussed in Chapter 1). While the state remains a powerful player in the regulation of healthcare, governmentality is premised on the principle of 'governing at a distance' through intermediary agencies. Since the state sponsors professions' self-regulatory status as a means of legitimizing their knowledge as expertise, these agencies are also subject to political governance in the interests of improving health outcomes in line with various policy goals such as cost rationalization, efficiency and efficacy. Evidence-based practice and management-led systems of clinical governance are two such emerging technologies, which are widely promoted within healthcare; the latter is seen as more politically controversial because it infringes on the self-regulatory domain of the medical profession (see Chapter 2 for further discussion). Both these technologies require new systems of knowledge and a new layer of regulatory agencies for the purposes of constructing and implementing standards. These strategies may be experienced in contradictory ways, in the way that both patient and professional agency is constrained and negotiated as discussed under the following themes:

- Changing relations between patients and health professionals;
- The tension between surveillance and empowerment;
- Negotiating relations of trust, knowledge and expertise;
- Governing the conduct of health professionals, and finally;
- The limits of neo-liberal policies of empowerment and participation.

Changing relations between patients and health professionals

Nettleton (1997) notes that as people are increasingly defined and invited to see themselves as autonomous agents in relation to their own health, the relationship between patients and experts changes. The patient or potential patient becomes a discerning consumer of the services and products that she invests in, and while subjectivity is increasingly bound up with expert knowledge, the expert's role is defined as advisory – providing information on how one can live a healthy life. In a series of earlier studies on how dental hygiene became part of the apparatus of governing health, Nettleton (1991, 1994) traces how dentistry sought new strategies for enrolling the support of mothers in the surveillance of their children's dental health. Initially, the target of dentistry was the individual patient who could be examined, monitored and trained in dental hygiene. To this end, mothers became the main target of dental health education (Nettleton 1991). Since disciplinary power concerns the production of expertise about norms of behaviour, the task of enrolling mothers in the promotion of their children's dental hygiene drew on the dominant ideology of Victorian motherhood to define dental health as an extension of women's realm of natural responsibility. Dental discourse incorporated a more psychological understanding of the patient when by the early twentieth century it had shifted its focus from treatment to prevention and monitoring. Dental knowledge has since extended its 'gaze' by emphasizing mothers' active health promotional role and seeking to understand the social contexts in which they can exercise such a role. In her interviews with mothers, Nettleton (1991) found that most had internalized this sense of responsibility and that they understand that the cost of resistance is that they may be held culpable for the dental status of their children's teeth and risk being seen as bad mothers. Rather than interpreting moral discourse as constraining or repressive in how mothers internalize disciplinary practices, Nettleton emphasizes the voluntary and promotional aspects of governmental technologies where mothers are constructed as active agents and health experts are cast as advisors. Nettleton's analysis follows Foucault's understanding of power as productive (discussed under the 'principles of poststructuralism'). Power is a productive force to the extent that it produces practical effects, for example, in producing a disciplined body whose capacity for health is maximized, and in that process it creates new fields of visibility, new targets, new discourses and practices and new modes of subjectivity or identity.

The tension between surveillance and empowerment

In a more recent study, Thompson (2008) posits a different kind of problem about the deployment of expert knowledge to promote individual
behaviour change. In examining the new and emerging role of the
Family Health Nurse (FHN) in New Zealand, she argues that the exercise
of biopower raises a central paradox for nurses in relation to the tension
between their surveillance role and the freedom implied by practices
that encourage individuals to govern themselves by adopting healthy
lifestyles. Indeed, Foucault's concept of biopower provokes a more critical reading of discourses of empowerment when deployed as a governmental strategy, which exposes the following paradox. On the one hand,
rather than involving constraining or repressive power, discourses of
empowerment (in the name of preventative health) operate primarily by
encouraging citizens to see themselves as self-governing. On the other
hand, governmentality may be viewed as producing more subtle and
intrusive forms of disciplinary power: the 'rational citizen' is one who
acquiesces to norms of behaviour consistent with expert knowledge.
Thompson argues that the new nursing role, which is defined by
the New Public Health Agenda as shifting health resources away from
curative medicine and hospital-based care to health promotion and
prevention in the community, is located in this tension or paradox.

A key role of the FHN concerns the incorporation of risk management into primary healthcare by carrying out a detailed family assessment over three generations to identify the prevalence of genetic risk
factors for the development of disease and to educate patients about
lifestyle changes to enable them to exert control over their own health
risks. As noted in Chapter 7, in the context of genetic medicine, the
patient is no longer someone who is sick but someone who is at risk of
developing a disease and the clinical focus shifts from the individual
patient to the family. The intrusive nature of this form of surveillance,
far from being seen as oppressive, acquires its meaning within the
nursing discourse of 'holism' and health promotion (imparting expert
information on individual family risk factors and advising on lifestyle
modifications).

Thompson, however, notes that the tension between surveillance and
empowerment places the FHN 'at the centre of governmentalising practices' where the potential to contribute to health gain is far from
straightforward. First, trust has to be built with patients to allow for such
intrusive surveillance about interpersonal relationships and lifestyle

choices and there is always the possibility of resistance. Second, it is difficult to measure health gains linked to lifestyle modification. These are not merely practical problems concerning individual motivation or technical problems of measurement. If subjects do not attach themselves to the project of health promotion and come to live their lives in accordance with expert knowledge, this is because of an inherent tension in governmentality between 'coercive power and civil liberties' (Thompson 2008: 77). In this sense, the jury is surely still out on whether health promotion is an effective strategy for producing a more positive knowledge relation to the self in a way that accords with the objectives of expert truths and the modes of possible action it promotes in terms of how we may exercise our autonomy. Since the liberal idea of the autonomous individual is the principle for rationalizing technologies of government, two elements come into play here in relation to governmental reason. The first is the legitimacy of specific techniques of government: the critical question here is whether the surveillance function associated with the role of the FHN encroaches upon the freedom of the subjects that it targets. The second element concerns the political and economic efficiency of its method: the question here is whether it can achieve its objective of health gain by encouraging individuals to manage their own health so that the economic and political cost to the state is less demanding. The tensions that emerge between risk surveillance and the promotion of individual autonomy for health professionals are further explored in relation to the case of child immunization below.

Negotiating relations of trust, knowledge and expertise

In the context of the delivery of healthcare, risk surveillance is intimately bound up with issues of trust and expertise. Following the public controversy surrounding the MMR vaccination and public health concerns about declining childhood immunization rates, the British government introduced a quota system for doctors to meet their vaccination targets. However, as Brownlie and Howson (2005) show, this only served to undermine public trust in doctors and expert knowledge. In a separate article Brownlie and Howson (2006) continue to explore this theme from the perspective of how primary care professionals engage with or resist governmental practices associated with child immunization programmes. They argue that in the wake of the MMR public controversy, an emerging characteristic of how health is governed is that knowledge and trust have become negotiable, in other words, the institutional authority that experts can claim and the trust that is a precondition of the exercise of that authority can no longer be taken for granted. They explore how target-setting linked to funding arrangements shapes practitioners' immunization practices and the implications this has for trust.

Brownlie and Howson (2006) found that both General Practitioners (GPs) and health visitors view target-setting for the uptake of MMR vaccination as problematic, particularly given that the new defaulters are middle-class, educated parents whose non-compliance is associated with heightened anxiety created by intense, negative media publicity. GPs generally fear that a perceived link between target-setting and financial incentives will undermine trust in their expertise, as well as limiting professional discretion in relation to the clinical management of individual cases. Health visitors, on the other hand, as front-line staff with responsibility for chasing up non-compliers and imparting information issued by the government, which some consider as biased, view their advocacy role as undermined. Brownlie and Howson make the point that in the immediate aftermath of intense media focus on Wakefield *et al.*'s (1998) paper, which suggested a causal link between the MMR vaccine and autism in children, health practitioners depended on government-sponsored information, which sought to downplay the uncertainties raised about the safety of the vaccination. This was seen as problematic in a climate where parents were actively taking up the policy mantle of the empowered consumer and 'expert patient' by accessing alternative sources of information and conflicting expert advice. Parental resistance was clearly not based on a lack of information and to construe it as a problem of misinformation risked undermining the apparent impartiality of health practitioners in relation to the emergence of a scientific knowledge dispute. For GPs and health visitors alike, there was a sense in which their expertise, clinical autonomy and respective roles were compromised by their dependence on state-sponsored information. As other studies show, public trust in government over its handling of this issue was low (Poltorak *et al.* 2005), as was public confidence in expertise (Casiday *et al.* 2006). Brownlie and Howson (2006: 441) conclude that the state's central role in the delivery of health services, which is reasserted through clinical governance, reinforces existing hierarchical relations of power where '...health visitors deliver targets for general practitioners who, in turn, deliver them for health managers'. This opens up new lines of tension that require health professionals to negotiate relations of trust, knowledge and expertise. From the perspective of public health, 'herd immunity' (Brownlie and Howson 2006: 434) is the best defence against population risk. However, there is a tension between clinical governance and the exercise of clinical discretion in individual cases that may undermine parents' trust in the objectivity of doctors.

The MMR controversy highlights a controversial aspect of Foucauldian analysis, namely its emphasis on how discourse *constitutes* the reality of bodies and bodily processes, which has been labelled by Bhaskar (1989) as the linguistic fallacy in that he contends it confuses existence with discourse about existence. Critical realists (see Chapter 5) criticize this position by arguing that it underplays the importance of criteria by which we can judge between different claims made about the body (Porter 1996a). The critical realist objection here is not to the observation that the nature of discourse surrounding diseases and their causation is of crucial importance, or that, in this instance, lay people's trust in health professionals was seriously eroded; rather it is that we need to realize that causes of disease exist (or do not exist) independently of discourse about them. While scientific evidence is certainly fallible (as attested by the fact that Wakefield *et al.*'s paper was accepted for publication by none other than the *Lancet*), critical realists argue that an acceptance that bodily reality is not simply constituted by discourse requires us to use critical judgement to weigh the evidence presented. At stake here is whether or not there are better and worse ways of knowing reality, and whether or not there are ways of adjudicating between them (Cheek and Porter 1997). However, as Layder notes,

> [Foucault] is not interested in whether the truth claims of discourses stand up to scrutiny. He is interested in the power effects of discourses which in themselves are neither true nor false. (Layder 1994: 105)

By revealing the contingent bases of knowledge, the relationship between knowledge and power appears less absolute and open to change (Delanty 1999). The idea that knowledge is socially constructed is further developed in Chapter 7 in relation to medical science and technology.

Governing the conduct of health professionals

Having discussed the challenges faced by health professionals in mediating scientific knowledge and public health targets in an audit culture, we return to Foucault's concept of governmentality as a theoretical framework for raising critical questions about how power operates in cultivating particular kinds of professional subjectivities. Using Foucault's theory of governmentality, Winch *et al.* (2002) show how evidence-based nursing constitutes an emerging form of governance that involves the political regulation of nursing, as well as cultivating a professional identity that socializes nurses into a scientific model of what constitutes nursing knowledge. The systematic review of research on nursing clinical practice renders nursing work visible in a quantitative way and, therefore, more open to interventions that set targets and standards for measuring the contribution of nursing care to healthcare service provision. As a technology of government, evidence-based nursing is premised on a positivist scientific paradigm, and Winch *et al.* contend,

> For those nurses (sic) researchers wishing to generate evidence with the capacity to influence health policy, the choice of knowledge-generating methods is increasingly clear; they either join the prevailing paradigm or become invisible. (2002: 159)

They also note that evidence-based practice not only enables interventions to set and monitor standards of nursing care in terms of what treatments work best, but it is also attractive as a policy framework to contain costs. They argue that the economic imperatives of the healthcare system impact directly on the arena of research. Since the randomized control trial is taken as the gold standard for generating evidence for clinical efficacy and since this is a resource-intensive methodology, Winch *et al.* speculate that research funding will be limited to those areas of clinical practices that are most costly to the state. At the same time, by investing in the authority of the scientific paradigm as a legitimate source of nursing knowledge, evidence-based practice has become an important political prong in the professionalization of nursing. However, the authors of this article also note that a considerable gap exists between the policy and academic currency afforded to evidence-based practice and its actual clinical implementation. To address this problem systematic reviews that focus on nurses' behaviour are now disseminated by nurse educators and administrators with a view to developing techniques for motivating nurses to put into practice evidence-based research. Nurses are not only expected to develop new skills and attitudes that embrace the scientific model of practice, but they have also become the objects of scientific knowledge aimed at promoting behavioural change amongst nurses. Winch *et al.* argue that the technologies of government associated with evidence-based practice have the potential to undermine nursing knowledge and identity based on what they call the 'intuitive experience of nursing', and to stymie a more critical kind of nursing knowledge. They observe in relation to the latter point:

> It is perhaps ironic that this type of approach [Foucault's concept of governmentality] and the sophisticated methods drawn from the more critical approaches of scholarly enquiry used by nurses have no place in the evidence-based practice movement. (Winch *et al.* 2002: 160)

It would seem particularly relevant at this point in the discussion to return to the empowerment strategies of neo-liberal health policies in relation to service users since this is often viewed as a strategy of the state to wrest power from healthcare professionals.

The limits of neo-liberal policies of empowerment and participation

Zibbel's (2004) study on drug policy treatment in Britain, which we discussed earlier, further explores the implications that arise from the neo-liberal construction of the drug user as an entrepreneurial subject by asking whether this shift in governmentality also involves a concomitant shift in the structural relations of power at the level of strategic decision-making concerning policy and the delivery of services. Zibbel's (2004: 62) analysis highlights the contradictory relations of power between what he terms 'welfare' and 'advanced liberal forms of governance'. The former is premised on the privilege of expert knowledge, which the state invests in as a form of authority that enables it to govern at a distance. The latter form of governance, on the other hand, invests in the governed subject as the 'expert' to be incorporated 'into a network of policy allegiances' (Zibbel 2004: 63). Zibbel's study shows that while a shift in technologies of governance gives some leverage to drug users to collectively demand a greater participatory role in strategic decision-making through policy and service consultation, this has little impact on the structural relations of power that govern the service user's relationship to professionals and policy makers who control resources and determine the terms of participation. In this respect, the author observes,

…an individual's sense of self is predicated on a relation to authority that provides the norms and conditions that define what kind of
behaviour is appropriate and what needs to be regulated. So, as drug
users become invested with expertise and participate in government
meetings they become governed not only by authorities, but also
through forms of self-policing in alignment with normative modes
of conduct (i.e. professionalism) dictated by their policy allegiances.
(Zibbel 2004: 63)

In this analysis, Zibbel is clearly pointing out that neo-liberal forms
of governmentality are not rationalized in terms of more democratic
forms of participation for the purpose of addressing structural relations
of inequality, but rather in making government more administratively
and politically efficient. Power relations appear far more stable than
governmentality studies sometimes lead us to believe; in deed, it would
appear that the leverage afforded by the liberal rhetoric of consumer
empowerment does little to contest or change professional power.

Conclusion and new directions for healthcare

Foucault is concerned with the micro-politics of power, most notably in
Discipline and Punish, where he details how the bodies and behaviours of
individuals and groups are marked, targeted, compared, categorized,
judged, examined and trained, and spatially distributed so that power can
operate through constant observation and surveillance. How Foucault
conceptualizes the operationalization of power and its relation to knowledge changes across his work. In *The Birth of the Clinic* power stems from a
particular field of visibility (e.g., the clinical gaze and the dominance this
affords medical discourse in defining the body and what constitutes
health). In *Discipline and Punish* power operates by shifting the focus of
control to the individual who is under surveillance and internalizes the
gaze of power, in other words, power is transformed into a subjectifying
or self-directing gaze. In *The History of Sexuality*, power operates by
encouraging individuals to become self-governing by means of practices
of the self (modes of subjectification derived from expert knowledge) so
that the objectives of government become seen as individual goals that
can be autonomously acted upon.

As we discussed in the opening section of this chapter, Foucault's
concepts of governmentality and biopower are closely related. He
argues that the capacity to sustain life and to incorporate the utility

of bodies into a productive and moral ideal of nation became a fundamental feature of modern society. Bio-power concerns the regulation of population and the disciplining of individual bodies, and governmentality refers to those strategies that are deployed to shape the conduct of populations not by constraining freedom but by regulating it through a complex assemblage of power relations connected to various modes of authority and expertise. The important point for Foucault is that practices of governing are not just about shoring up the sovereign power of the state, but of 'governing at a distance' through a wide range of agencies. These agencies exercise their authority through various technologies to promote not only, for example, health, but also modes of self-government that experts have identified as serving such ends. Governmentality assumes its liberal form through technologies that simultaneously promote self-government.

In line with Foucault's concern with technologies of self in his later work and his theory of governmentality, contemporary studies tend to emphasize changing relations between the two poles of biopower where the balance is tipped over from technologies of power (domination) to technologies of self. It is difficult to escape interpreting this transformation in governmentality as simply a more insidious way of governing and perfecting a more subtle form of power that is imperceptible to those who are governed and, hence, making power all the more effective without threatening the sovereign power of the state (e.g., to minimize its sphere of responsibility, to divert the cost of health to market forces, or more worryingly, to limit its duty of care to those who fail to fulfil the obligation of taking responsibility for their health in ways consistent with expert knowledge) and the authority it invests in experts to govern from a distance. While Foucault understood that resistance is part of the dynamics of power, in his early work individuals appear as mere docile bodies enveloped by a deterministic, subjugating and normalizing power, and subject to the imposition of dominant discourses such as medicine. Both his concept of governmentality and his emphasis on technologies of the self in the last two volumes of *The History of Sexuality* (1985, 1986) led Foucault to emphasize the agency of the individual subject. So instead of viewing subjectivity as an effect of the imposition of discourses enacted through technologies of domination, Foucault begins to emphasize individual agency or autonomy in terms of the interrelationship between technologies of domination (the imperative of surveillance at the institutional level) and practices of the self (those practices that enable individuals to engage in the conduct of their own lives). However, the disjuncture between Foucault's earlier and later work leads to contradictions resulting in what Armstrong (1997) sees as very different interpretations of Foucault's work (see also Fox 1997, Lupton 1997).

The empirical research that we discuss in the second half of the chapter applies Foucault's concept of governmentality to trace the changes that are occurring in the relations of knowledge, power and expertise that govern health. Furthermore, they link the governance of health to wider political rationales as a way of explaining how the reconfiguration of health policy and the emergence of new technologies such as health promotion construct particular modes of subjectivity at both the individual and the collective level. Most of these studies address the implications of a prevailing neo-liberal rationality on healthcare, while others identify tensions and ambiguities that are emergent or manifest and that raise questions for further research about the future of healthcare. In particular, more recent studies such as Winch *et al.* (2002), Brownlie and Howson (2006) and Thompson (2008) demonstrate how Foucault's ideas can be applied to more critical readings of how health professionals mediate the way that governmentality seeks to articulate technologies of power with technologies of self; and in the case of the first two studies, respectively, the implications that clinical governance holds for healthcare knowledge and practice, and the formative role that it can play in shaping the relationship between trust and expertise.

As a critical theory, poststructuralism opens up new perspectives that question different facets of health and healthcare that have hitherto been taken for granted or assumed unproblematic. For example, if care is reconceptualized in terms of the exercise of power, we are led to reconsider the values that we assume are expressed in the theories and practice of care. Equally, this same framework challenges discourses of empowerment as having the opposite effect of oppressive practices, and maybe viewed as producing more subtle forms of disciplinary power expressed by the principles of 'self-care' and 'self-responsibilization'. At the same time, as we come to live our lives and construct our identities on the basis of the personal freedoms implied by the choices surrounding the commodification of health and the understanding that health is within our control as autonomous and rational subjects, new modes of resistance emerge and the relationship between patients and health professionals increasingly becomes negotiable. As responsibility for health shifts from the state to the individual, the relationship between health professionals and patients and the realm of personal freedom is regulated by the state through clinical governance. Therefore, the construction of the patient as 'consumer' and 'expert' (e.g., patient charters and patient consumer panels to guide service delivery and health policy) coupled with strategies for standardizing and regulating healthcare practices (e.g., target setting linked to funding arrangements or evidence-based practice linked to the standardization of knowledge) derive their value as an administrative strategy to make government more administratively and politically efficient. The principle of responsibilization and the contesting ethical and political expectations it creates in relation to health suggests a fruitful research agenda in terms of a more critical approach to neo-liberal healthcare policies.

CHAPTER 5

Critical Realism, Health and Healthcare

Introduction

Critical realism is a broad philosophy. It addresses ontology – questions concerning what exists, epistemology – questions concerning what we can know about what exists, and ethics – what we should do about what we discover exists. Critical realism's concerns are, like Science and Technology Studies (see Chapter 7), wider than those of social theory, in that it also addresses questions about the natural world. Because all of these issues link together within the critical realist model, it will be necessary to stray a bit beyond the strict parameters of social theory in order to give the reader a clear idea of critical realism in the round.

In general terms, critical realism, as formulated in the work of the contemporary British philosopher, Roy Bhaskar, might be described as an alternative way of looking at things to the two main poles of social theory. It rejects both the notion that human behaviour is governed by deterministic social laws (as espoused by structural functionalism, described in Chapter 1) and it equally rejects the assumption that individual interpretation and interaction is the appropriate focus for sociology (for a position close to this, see Chapter 2 on social interaction theory). This alternative perspective in the debate about the relative importance of social structure or social action informs critical realism's views about how we should approach the social world, in that it equally rejects positivist attempts to discover invariable relations in the social world and postmodernist scepticism about the possibility of uncovering empirically any sort of generalizable information. The 'critical' bit in critical realism is where ethics comes in, in that the point of social knowledge from this perspective is to discover that which enables or restrains human freedom, happiness and fulfilment. In other words, critical realism does not claim to be value neutral – it sees itself as a social theory that can be used to critically analyse social relationships in order to expose inequalities and the factors that promote them.

As with other chapters, this one begins by looking at the principles of critical realism, beginning with general principles of what exists and how causal relations work, and then moving on to examine what it has to say about the social world, and in particular, its position on the structure/agency controversy mentioned above. The final principle to be discussed is the critical part of critical realism. In the section on understanding health, we take three examples, namely Peter Conrad's (1999) critique of simplistic views of genetics, Simon Williams' contribution to the disability debate and Graham Scambler's (2001) discussion of sociological explanations of inequalities in health. Finally, in looking at how critical realism might help us understand healthcare, we examine the use of realist evaluation methods to explain the success and failure of complex healthcare interventions. These methods go beyond simply evaluating the intervention itself and try to explain the processes involved between its introduction and the outcomes that are produced.

Principles of critical realism

What exists?

At its most general level, the philosophical position of realism involves the assumption that there is an external reality, independent of our experiences of it or our thoughts about it. In other words, it assumes that knowledge, in general, and science, in particular, is about something. This position can be contrasted with that of idealism (used in its philosophical rather than general sense), which argues that we have no evidence that anything exists outside of our thoughts and perceptions. The debate between realism and idealism is the sort of conundrum that can go round and round for ever without coming to a definitive conclusion. However, for the sake of argument, we might accept the most famous realist attempt to short-circuit this debate – Samuel Johnson's response to the great Irish idealist, George

Berkeley (for whom the University of California campus is named), as recounted by Boswell:

> After we came out of the church, we stood talking for some time together of Bishop Berkeley's ingenious sophistry to prove the non-existence of matter, and that everything in the universe is merely ideal. I observed, that though we are satisfied his doctrine is not true, it is impossible to refute it. I never shall forget the alacrity with which Johnson answered, striking his foot with mighty force against a large stone, till he rebounded from it – "I refute it *thus*." (Boswell 1998: 333)

Working from this general realist foundation, the critical realist philosopher Roy Bhaskar (1989a) interrogates reality further, arguing that it consists of three levels. The first level he terms the empirical. This consists of events that are experienced by humans. The second level, the actual, consists of all events, whether experienced or not. Here we come back to the assertion of reality outside our perception of it. In terms of that hoary old riddle, when a tree falls in the forest when there is no one around, it does make a sound. The third level of reality does not relate to events at all, but to the forces that cause those events to happen. These mechanisms are not even potentially the objects of direct experience, so how can they be regarded as real? Bhaskar (1978) argues that they should be seen as such because they satisfy what he terms the causal criterion for reality – they are real because they cause events to occur.

Let us take an example of leaves falling from a tree in autumn. If we stand and watch an oak tree on a windy day, we will observe great numbers of its leaves floating to the ground – this is an empirical event. If we wander inside to get out of the wind, we can be confident that the leaves will not cease falling from the tree – this is an actual event. However, we need to ask why are we so confident that the leaves keep falling when we are not there to witness them. We do this by resorting to the third level of reality, the causal, which provides us with an explanation as to *why* they should fall. Leaves fall to the earth rather than floating up into the sky because they are subject to gravitational force. Gravity is not something that we can see or feel, but we experience its effects all around us. The fact that it can cause these observable effects is proof of its reality.

You might think this a rather simplistic example, and indeed it is. All leaves on trees are subject to gravity, but not all leaves fall to the earth.

Other mechanisms need to be in operation as well. In the example, we noted it was a windy day; this is significant in that it is the mechanical force of the wind against the leaves that helps pull them away from the tree. In turn, the wind is caused by the pressure gradient force. Yet, you might say, even in the strongest of winds, many trees hold on to their leaves. We must also add to the explanation the process of abscission, whereby physiological changes in deciduous plants lead to a weakening of the connection between leaf and plant in autumn.

Causality

We use the above example to illustrate how critical realism's conception of causality differs from standard notions of cause and effect that rely on the identification of what is termed 'constant conjunction'. This term was coined by the eighteenth-century Scottish philosopher, David Hume ([1739–1740] 1969), who argued that the way we identify causal laws is by experiencing one event occurring immediately after another over and over again. Thus, for Hume the way we identify the law of gravity is by observing that every time we drop something, it falls to the ground – there is a constant conjunction between dropping and falling.

Positivist science is to a large degree predicated upon the assumption of constant conjunction. Thus, the classic experiment seeks to identify a solid relationship between a cause and effect by isolating a relationship of constant conjunction between the independent variable and the dependent variable, with all other known potential sources of variation controlled. In other words, a closed system is created in order to clarify the relationship between dependent and independent variables.

The problem here is that closed systems are artificial constructs – events normally occur in open systems, in which a number of causal mechanisms may be operating at the same time, some reinforcing the effects of each other and some countervailing them. To return to trees and leaves, it can be seen that pressure gradient and gravitational forces mutually reinforce the tendency for leaves to drop, and when they are combined with the internal process of abscission, it is likely that the tree will shed its leaves. However, if the tree happens to be an evergreen, the absence of a genetic trigger for abscission means that the leaves are unlikely to fall. In short, causal relations in open systems do not involve constant conjunction between a determinist cause and its effect, but instead consist of complex interactions between a number of causal forces, whose precise relationship will differ from context to context. It is on these grounds that Bhaskar argues that causal mechanisms should be regarded as tendencies, stating that 'in citing a law one is referring to the...activity of a mechanism...not making a claim about the actual outcome (which in general will be co-determined by the activity of other mechanisms)' (Bhaskar 1989a: 9–10).

While the nature of open systems makes it unlikely that invariant regularities will obtain within them, the existence of causative tendencies means that there are likely to be partial regularities. Lawson (1997) terms this type of event as a demi-regularity, or demi-reg, which he defines as:

> A partial event regularity which *prima facie* indicates the occasional, but less than universal, actualisation of a mechanism or tendency... The patterning observed will not be strict if countervailing factors sometimes dominate or frequently co-determine the outcomes in a variable manner. But where demi-regs are observed, there is evidence of relatively enduring and identifiable tendencies in play. (Lawson 1997: 204)

The social world

The fact that the discussion has centred around trees and leaves thus far may be causing you some concern, given that we are meant to be addressing people. In answer to this concern, it is time to point out that critical realism claims that its tenets can be applied to the social world as well as the natural. The first thing to note is that people's actions are not random, their behaviour has patterns. While these patterns are not invariable, but are demi-regular, their existence implies that there is more governing human action than isolated individual motivation. This is not to deny the importance of individuals' decision-making capacities, merely to point out that, on their own, they cannot explain the regularities and commonalities of behaviour they display. Critical realism argues that an adequate explanation of human action has to include consideration of the social structures that influence those actions. Note the use of the word 'influence', rather than 'determine'. Critical realism does not subscribe to hard line structuralist views of humans which see them as automatons responding automatically to the dictates of social structures. For one thing, society is an extremely complex open system, in which there are many structures operating simultaneously, some reinforcing and some contradicting each other. But it is not just a matter of social complexity. We also need to take account of the influences upon our behaviour that emanate from our individual psychology and biology, including our genetic dispositions. When all of these are taken into account, it becomes clear that the capacity to totally explain, still less predict, the actions of particular individuals is not possible. For critical realism, the aim of the social scientist is to identify the tendencies generated by social structures.

Social structures

At this point, you may well still have concerns about the emphasis on the natural world and the apparent espousal by critical realism of the philosophical position of naturalism – the doctrine that because the social world is essentially the same as the natural world, it is amenable to the same methods of investigation as those used to understand nature. The problem here is that, in contrast to natural structures such as gravity or magnetism, social structures are not independent entities; their existence depends upon the actions of individuals. For example, the structured relations involved in marriage only exist because people choose to get married and would cease to exist if they chose otherwise. Bhaskar (1989a) notes this crucial distinction and identifies it as a significant limitation to the possibility of naturalism as the basis for social science.

As the example of marriage implies, critical realism has a clear conception of the nature of social structures – they consist of persistent relations between individuals and groups (Bhaskar 1989a). All our social attributes imply a social relationship. For example, we are only a nurse, doctor or physiotherapist by dint of our relationship with patients; we are only a worker because of our relationship with our employers and so on. Of course, it is more complicated than this. For example, the social position of being a nurse also involves nurses' relationships with physicians and other healthcare workers. There is thus a lattice-work of relations that forms the structure of society, and it is this structure of relations, according to critical realists, which constitutes the appropriate subject matter of social science (Collier 1994). This relational conception of society can be summed up using the words of Karl Marx (1973a [1857–1858]: 265): 'Society does not consist of individuals, but expresses the sum of interrelations, the relations within which these individuals stand.'

Structure and agency

Critical realism's relational theory of society leads to a further issue, namely the need for it to provide an adequate explanation for this seemingly circular relationship between social structure and individual agency whereby both appear to influence each other. Probably the best-known contemporary attempt to deal with the relationship between structure and agency has been Anthony Giddens' (1976) structuration theory, which seeks 'to explain how it comes about that structures are constituted through action, and reciprocally how action is constituted structurally' (1976: 161). In rejecting both structuralist arguments that social actions are determined by social structures and interpretivist arguments (see Chapter 3) that they are entirely the result of individual motivation, Giddens (1976) argues that structure and agency are two sides of the same coin. While structures provide the rules and resources to enable individual social actors to behave in the ways that they do, those rules and resources have only a virtual existence until they are 'instantiated' (brought into existence) through social actions. To go back to the example of patterns of domestic cohabitation, up until well into the twentieth century the nature of gendered relations in Western societies meant that the overwhelming norm for young adults was to enter a heterosexual marriage, thus human action was structured in a very particular way. However, the structure of marriage only exists in so far as people decide to actually get married. As we have seen in recent decades across many Western countries, fewer and fewer people are deciding to instantiate marriage, thus weakening its structural influence as a social norm.

While having much in common with structuration theory, critical realism differs in that it sees structure and action as separate entities rather than as two sides of the same coin. If structures only have a virtual existence until they are instantiated by social actions, this leads to the paradox of structures coming into existence at the same moment as the actions that they condition. This is not merely a philosophical quibble. As Margaret Archer points out, it means that 'structuration theory cannot recognize that structure and agency work on different time intervals' (1995: 89). While accepting Giddens' (1976) point that social structures cannot exist independently of social actions, Archer (1995) asks the question: 'whose actions?' Her answer is based on Auguste Comte's aphorism that the majority of actors are the dead. The social structures that influence our lives have not been conjured up by our instantiation of them. Instead, they are the result of previous actions. Thus, they have an existence prior to our experience of them. Think, for example, of the English language, which involves a particular structure of communication developed long ago by our ancestors, into which we are introduced in our early years. However, while we do not create structures through our actions, those actions either maintain or transform pre-existing structures. To return to language, to the extent that it remains in a form that would be recognizable to our ancestors, we are maintaining it through our usage. To the extent that it evolves and develops through the introduction of new words and grammatical structures, we are transforming it.

It should be noted that transforming social structures is a considerably more arduous and slower process than Giddens' notion of instantiation would suggest. There are two main reasons for inertia in structural change. First, not everyone will want to change things – there will be many who benefit from the old ways and want to stick to them. Second, the structural conditions pertaining often place limitations on the speed of change.

Take the example of childbirth. In recent years there has been a general movement to structure childbirth services in a new way – to move away from highly medicalized care located on hospital wards. However, despite evidence to support the efficacy of this re-structuring, in terms of both clinical outcomes and the experiences of those receiving care, the move away from physician-led hospital-based childbirth services has been disappointingly slow. Why should this be? Well, first we might look to an extremely powerful social group in whose interests it is to maintain the status quo, namely obstetricians. Second, the way maternity care has been structured in Western countries for so long means that few midwives have sufficient experience of independent practice to be able to take on the responsibilities that the new modes of care would require. This in turn means there are few midwifery educationalists capable of teaching these skills, which further delays the recruitment of sufficient numbers of appropriately skilled midwives. So, even if there were no opposition to these reforms, there would still be a considerable lapse between policy decisions to promote choice in childbirth and the development of structures to facilitate such a choice.

The realist view of the relationship between structure and agency is probably most succinctly and indeed poetically summed up using the words of Karl Marx ([1852] 1973b: 146):

Men [sic] make their own history, but...not under circumstances they themselves have chosen but under the given and inherited circumstances with which they are directly confronted. The tradition of the dead generations weighs like a nightmare on the minds of the living.

Examining structure and agency

Having discussed critical realism's ontology of society – what it states exists, it is time now to look at the strategies critical realists use to find out about what exists (their epistemology). The first thing to note is that they have a big problem in terms of the admitted fact that structures are not amenable to direct observation; they can only be detected by means of their effects. In other words, structured social relationships are not things that can be directly perceived, but can only be inferred from the actions that they influence.

This may seem like an almost insurmountable problem, but it is one that all of us surmount in our everyday interpretations of the world. We will take a historical example, the Los Angeles 'Rodney King' riots of 1992, which involved thousands of Afro-Americans. The riots were triggered by the verdict of a predominantly white jury, which acquitted four white police officers of using excessive force in the arrest of Rodney King, who was black, despite graphic and widely seen video footage of them assaulting King with truncheons and tasers. Thus, the Afro-American population of Los Angeles were confronted with two sets of actions – one involving white policemen severely beating a black man and the other involving a predominantly white jury deciding to acquit those policemen despite widely disseminated evidence of their brutal actions. Their interpretation of what lay behind these events – what led them to occur – was a deeply racist society in which oppressive social relations were so pernicious that they had infected the judicial system to the core. In other words, people did not riot simply because some individuals got off with beating up another individual; they rioted because they regarded those actions as providing clear evidence that the structure of the society in which they lived meant that they could not expect protection under the rule of law and that the only way to alter that structure was to take the law into their own hands.

Leaving aside the rights and wrongs of rioting, the main point here is that the process of interpretation used by those who rioted (and many more besides) involved moving from experience of particular actions to positing the conditions which led to those actions. This is precisely the form of logic used by critical realism, which involves applying what is termed, following the German Enlightenment philosopher Immanuel Kant ([1781] 1907), the 'transcendental question', namely asking: 'what must be the case in order for events to occur as they do?' (Porter 2001).

Once again, it can be seen that critical realism adopts an alternative strategy to the two main approaches to generating scientific knowledge. Rather than choosing between deduction – inferring from the general to the particular, or induction – inferring from the particular to the general, critical realism uses what is termed 'retroduction' – inferring 'from a description of some phenomenon to a description of something which produces it or is a condition for it' (Bhaskar 1986: 11).

While critical realism adheres to a clear view of the general strategy that should be used to gain knowledge of underlying structures, namely retroductive analysis, it is less prescriptive about the particular methods that should be adopted within this strategy. However, the general principles as outlined above tend to provide implicit support for the use of a mixed methods approaches (McEvoy and Richards 2006). Regularities and patterns of actions and interactions are best uncovered using quantitative methods, while the motivations behind those actions and interactions require the use of qualitative methods; as Bhaskar (1989a) observes, meanings cannot be measured, only understood.

The critical approach

We have seen that the aim of critical realism when applied to the analysis of society is to uncover the structured relations that generate the patterns of interaction that take place between people. For critical realists, this is not simply an academic exercise. Critical exposure of structured relations and the restraints and enablements they place on people's ability to act in their own interests has practical consequences in that such information can be used to inform attempts to improve the structural organization of society, reinforcing those types of structured relationship that enhance human freedom and dignity, and minimizing those that inhibit it (Bhaskar 1989b). Here we come back to the relationship between agency and structure, whereby it is possible for actors to either maintain or transform the structures with which they are confronted. Critical realism aspires to provide intellectual ammunition for the transformation of oppressive structures. Once again, there is no better a person to sum up this critical approach to intellectual labour than Karl Marx: (1974 [1888]: XI) 'The philosophers have only *interpreted* the world, in various ways; the point is to *change* it.' However, it is important not to get too carried away with the possibilities of critical knowledge. As Bhaskar puts it:

> To be free is (i) to know, (ii) to possess the opportunity and (iii) to be disposed to act in (or towards) one's real interests...*[E]mancipation*...is both *causally presaged* and *logically entailed* by explanatory theory, but...can only be effected in *practice*. (1989b: 89–90)

Before moving on to the next section, we should explain our repeated use of quotations from Karl Marx. For critical realists such as Bhaskar (1989b), Marx's ideas, with their characterization of society structured and moulded by enduring relations, and belief in the transformational capacity of social action, provide an early example of critical realism, albeit one that privileges the relations of production as determining other aspects of social life (see Chapter 1 also). While contemporary realists tend to regard assertions that everything can be explained in terms of economic relations as too limiting in that they fail to give due account to the influence of other structured relations, such as those of race or ethnicity, the general thrust of Marx's ideas remain pertinent, as we hope the quotations used here demonstrate. That said we should point out that while Marx was a realist, and while most critical realists would accept that economic relations are an important facet of the structure of society, you do not have to follow Marxism in all its details to be a critical realist.

Applications to understandings of health

Given the broadness of critical realism's approach and claims to explanatory usefulness, there are all sorts of examples that could be used in relation to health (and illness) to explore how it might illuminate an issue. What we wish to do here is concentrate on just three topics that address the causes of health and illness and disability. The first example looks at the doctrine of specific aetiology, focusing on Peter Conrad's (1999) critique of its application to genetics. While Conrad does not adopt a critical realist approach, we have chosen his paper as a point of discussion because it illustrates nicely how the problems he identifies in relation to causation are amenable to a critical realist explanation. The second example looks at how we understand disability, drawing on Simon Williams' (1999) argument that an adequate understanding requires us to take account of both biology and society. The third example involves Graham Scambler's (2001a) discussion of sociological explanations of inequalities in health. In this paper, Scambler explicitly applies critical realism to the debate. Once again, his concern is how the realist position can improve our understanding of the causal processes involved in generating inequalities of health.

'The mirage of genes'

Conrad's (1999) critique of popular (and to some degree medical) conceptions of genetics is grounded in the seminal work of Rene Dubos (1959). One of Dubos' prime targets was germ theory, the notion that microbes cause disease. Dubos identified two main assumptions of germ theory. The first was the doctrine of specific aetiology, which states that every disease has a specific cause, and, in relation to infectious diseases, that the specific cause will be a microbe, either bacterial or viral. The second, related assumption involved attributing primary importance to the internal as opposed to the external environment. In terms of clinical understanding of diseases, the focus of attention was on how microbes affected cells, tissues and organs to produce disease. The individual's relationship to the outside environment became a secondary issue.

Taking the example of the history of tuberculosis, Dubos noted that mortality rates from the disease were declining even before Koch had identified the tubercle bacillus, never mind the introduction of chemotherapy in the form of streptomycin. Conversely, he noted that many individuals who were infected by the bacillus did not display the disease. This led him to argue that germ theory was simplistic, and at times misleading. In contrast to the doctrine of specific aetiology, he argued that while germs were necessary causes of infectious diseases (in other words, you could not get tuberculosis if you were not infected by the tubercle bacillus), they were not sufficient, in that other factors needed to be taken into account. Many of those factors, such as access to adequate nutrition, were to be found in the external environment.

Conrad (1999) brings the story up to date by arguing that genes are the new germs, and that, while the focus has shifted from one to the other, the same misleading notions of disease causation remain. In terms of specific aetiology, we now have a monogenic model of disease causation, whereby a gene or genetic mutation is regarded as determining a disease or behaviour. Moreover, the focus on DNA is, by definition, a focus on the internal environment. Thus, for example, genes rather than cultural meanings of drinking are seen as the cause of alcoholism. As Conrad puts it, with the genetic version of specific aetiology, 'nature trumps nurture' (1999: 231). While it should be admitted that in a number of cases, such as cystic fibrosis, nature does indeed trump nurture, in that the presence of a single gene causes the disease, these are relatively rare. In the vast majority of cases 'genes are not directly deterministic, if we mean that if the gene is present an individual will inevitably get the disorder...For most diseases...genes are a probabilistic rather than deterministic cause' (1999: 233). On a similar line, Rose argues that the application of the doctrine of specific aetiology to the new genetics 'disarticulates complex properties of individuals into isolated lumps of biology' (1995: 381).

In terms of the relationship between the internal and the external environments – nature and nurture – Conrad points out that the problem is not simply one of underestimating the importance of the environment in which genetic tendencies are expressed. It is also a matter of failing to grasp the complex causal relationship that exists between nature and nurture. He quotes Lewontin (1991: 30) to make the point:

Environmental variation and genetic variation are not independent causal pathways. Genes affect how sensitive one is to the environment and environment affects how relevant one's genetic differences may be.

All in all, Conrad's (1999) critique of the new genetics, or at least the popular and medical understandings of it, is fairly damning. Just as germ theory before it, its notions of simple causations that occur within our bodies are dangerously misleading in that they pull the focus of health maintenance and disease prevention away from the many social and environmental factors that are crucial in the development and prevalence of many diseases and which are amenable to change given sufficient resources and political will. So what is the way forward? Unfortunately, Conrad is rather pessimistic in his prognosis about the rise of the new germ theory:

> Perhaps the fate of genetic explanations will parallel that of germ theory; decontextualising aetiological processes, underrepresenting the role of environments, producing some stunning medical interventions, revealing little about the fate of populations, and becoming the most popular explanation for what ails us. The rising influence and ubiquity of the genetic paradigm is already evident in medicine and popular discourse. It is our challenge to continue to explicate the social realities of illness and behaviour in the midst of an enticing and widening genetic mirage. (Conrad 1999: 239–240)

From a critical realist perspective, a major part of the problem here is the notion of causality that underlies the doctrine of specific aetiology. It is unsurprising that this doctrine enjoys such widespread acceptance in that it fits in so easily with the positivist conception of causality as constant conjunction. In turn, the inadequacies of explanation and the consequent distortion of responses to disease highlight the weaknesses in the positivist model of causality. In contrast, the realist conception of causes as tendencies whose interaction with other tendencies will co-determine outcomes provides a causal model that is better able to take account of the complex interaction of factors. Moreover, critical realism's insistence that human beings (including their bodies) exist in multiple open systems, including biological, psychological and social systems, and that tendencies from all these systems need to be taken into account allows us to overcome the false dichotomy between internal and external environments. Finally, in terms of the critical aspect of critical realism, it can be seen how it can provide the basis for a critique of the technocentrism of these approaches to health and illness which reduce them to technical problems that are soluble through the actions of experts, be they physicians or geneticists. By emphasizing the more contingent social factors in the aetiology of disease, critical realism has the potential to provide knowledge that can be used for action to improve the health of the population.

Disabled bodies or societies?

It might be concluded from the above example of genetics that the main thrust of critical realism in understanding health, illness and disability is to emphasize social structure. However, it has also been used to counter-balance what critical realists regard as one-sided social approaches. This is the case in Williams' response to the social model of disability.

In opposition to the medical model of disability which emphasizes its bodily basis, those who adhere to the social model of disability argue that it is a purely social phenomenon. Rather than being the result of physical impairment, disability is a form of social oppression (Oliver 1990). From this perspective, the body has nothing to do with disability, which instead is the result of social prejudices and barriers that prevent those classed as disabled participating in society on equal terms (Swain *et al.* 1993). It is easy to see why this approach has been attractive to disability activists in that it moves disability away from being a medical problem, whereby the medical profession has a monopoly over defining disability and prescribing what should be done about it, and places it onto the terrain of human rights, enabling disabled people to fight on their own terms the very real discrimination to which they are subjected. However, there is a major problem with such an approach – making society everything and writing the body out of the story may de-medicalize disability, but it does so at the cost of allowing the medical approach to monopolize understandings of the impaired body. In other words, it does not effectively challenge the biomedical monopoly over knowledge about the body (Hughes and Patterson 1997).

This is where critical realism comes in. From this perspective, disability emerges from the complex interactions of biological, social and cultural structures, and as a result cannot be fully understood by recourse to any one of these factors on their own (Williams 1999). While accepting the importance of the body in understanding disability, critical realism's assertion that social structures are subject to transformation through people's actions, both individually and collectively, enables it to be used as a basis for political activism. In other words, it overcomes the problems of both bio-medical and social reductionism, while still maintaining the promise of change. As Williams (1999: 812–813) puts it:

> The critical realist approach...enables us to: (i) bring the biological body, impaired or otherwise, 'back in'; (ii) relate the individual to society in a challenging...way, and; (iii) rethink questions of identity,

difference and the ethics of care through a commitment to real bodies and real selves, real lives and real worlds'

Rather than peeling off society from the body and thus allowing the biomedical paradigm to maintain its monopoly over the latter, by insisting on the interaction between biological and social structures in its conception of disability, critical realism provides at least the promise of introducing more democratic discourses into conceptions of bodily impairments and how these articulate with social oppression.

Inequalities in health

The third example we wish to discuss is Graham Scambler's critique of sociological explanations of health inequalities, which involves an extension of the arguments examined in Chapters 1 and 2. Scambler accuses sociological research on health inequalities, especially that relating to social class, of lacking sociological imagination. The reasons for this are grounded in the familiar problem of a commitment to positivist methodologies with their conception of regularities of constant conjunction. This is reinforced by the influence of social epidemiology, at whose core lies the analysis of regular associations. All this results in 'a stultifying lack of interest in generative mechanisms' (Scambler 2001a: 35).

The first thing to look at is how social class is defined. In the copious literature on health inequalities, from the seminal Black Report (Townsend *et al.* 1992) through the Registrar General's measure of occupational class (RGOC) to the current National Statistics Socio-Economic Classification (NS-SEC) (Office for National Statistics 2002) in Britain, and socio-economic status (SES) in the United States, a common approach can be detected. The different 'classes' into which these systems divide people are essentially proxies for the life chances that people enjoy, whether those life chances are attained by income from property or employment salary. At the top are the better paid jobs with higher status, with remuneration and status decreasing as we go down the class grades. Put another way, they involve a rejection of the Marxist definition of class which is structured according to the relations of production, with the great class fissure being drawn between those who own and control the means of production (the bourgeoisie) and those who do not but who labour to produce the wealth for those who do (the proletariat). Instead, they accept the Weberian definition of class, which includes three criteria:

1. 'a number of people have in common a specific causal component of their life chances' (Weber 1970: 181) – a group of people whose circumstances provide them with similar access to goods and services and living conditions.
2. 'this component is represented exclusively by economic interests in the possession of goods and opportunities for income' (Weber 1970: 181) – class relates to the degree of economic power that different groups have to access the good life.
3. 'is represented under the conditions of the commodity or labour markets' (Weber 1970: 181) – rather than just two opposing classes, there are a plurality of groups competing in the market where goods and services are exchanged at a price. While the ownership of property confers considerable advantage, it is not the only source of economic power in the market.

One of the main arguments for the rejection of the Marxist definition of class for the measurement of class inequalities is that within the proletariat (which constitutes the vast majority of people) there are such huge differences in status and income that lumping them all together provides far too crude an instrument for measuring inequalities (Parkin 1979). As we shall see, critical realists (and Marxists) argue that this is to miss the point.

To sum up the findings of the British literature on inequalities of health to which Scambler largely refers, there has been a consistent correlation between higher occupational class and higher health chances in terms of mortality and morbidity, and for a considerable period of time now, despite an overall increase in life expectancy, these inequalities in health have been widening (see, e.g., the Acheson Report, Stationary Office 1998). An interesting variation on these findings that relies on the same positivist methodological principles is provided by Wilkinson (1996), who argues that once a society reaches a certain level of Gross National Product (GNP), the principle determinant of health chances is not the level of income people have, but the degree of inequality that pertains within their society. He argues that this is because increased social inequality leads to reduced social cohesion and trust, resulting in a hostile and inhospitable environment for those facing the brunt of inequality (Wilkinson 1999).

We have already discussed the strengths and weaknesses of Wilkinson's position in Chapters 1 and 2. However, even if we accept that his argument is empirically correct, Scambler argues that it does not go far enough. Crucially, it cannot explain what causes the poverty and social inequality that lead to inequalities in health. In critical realist terms, this approach concentrates exclusively on the demi-regularities (Lawson 1997) of association between poverty/social inequality and inequalities in health, but fails to uncover the underlying mechanisms which generate those demi-regularities. In Scambler's words, the search for causes is called off too early. This is where the failure of the sociological imagination is manifest – if the causes of this sorry state of affairs are not identified, then the capacity to transform society in such a way that reduces inequalities in health is fatally compromised. That this may well be the case is evidenced by the fact that, despite vast amounts of epidemiological evidence about demi-regular associations, health inequalities continue to widen.

For Scambler (2001a), a full understanding of what is going on requires us to take into account the structured economic relations that generate the demi-regularities that we observe, and for him, the best model of those relations is provided by the Marxist conception of the relations of production. He argues that this is a relationship between three primary groups – members of the 'capital-executive' whose ownership of the means of production enables them to command strategic economic decision-making; members of the new middle class (including those who run the state), who regulate the economy through tactical decision-making; and those who participate in, or co-ordinate, the labour process, who belong to a collective labour class. For those in the first two groups, the logic of capital accumulation is paramount.

On the basis of these observations, Scambler formulates his colourfully named 'greedy bastards hypothesis' which 'states that Britain's enduring, widening health inequalities might reasonably be regarded as the (largely unintended) consequences of the ever-adaptive behaviours of members of its…power elite, informed by its…capital-executive' (2001a: 39). Thus, economic deregulation, the dismantling of state influence in 'command economies' and the de-standardization of work which are the results of strategic decisions to increase capital accumulation have in turn resulted in increases in social inequalities which in turn have led to increases in health inequalities.

It can be seen that, in this example, because we are dealing with an economic problem, critical realism takes on a neo-Marxist guise. It is those structured relations revolving round the production of goods and services and the profits to be made from them that provide the mechanisms to generate economic inequalities. In a way, if correct, this analysis is a rather depressing one, in that it could be argued that if health inequalities are the consequence of contemporary capitalism, then the chances of actually being able to do anything significant about them are slim. After all, as Bhaskar observed earlier, it is not simply a matter of understanding the problems we are faced with, but also having the opportunity to act on them. Nevertheless, it provides a good example of how critical realism attempts to delve deeper into the reasons behind observed conditions and events, in contrast to conventional positivist science that is often content to simply describe those conditions and events. Here we can see clearly the critical nature of the enterprise, its point being not simply to describe health inequalities, but to change them.

Applications to understandings of healthcare

In our application of critical realism as an aid to understanding healthcare, we are going to concentrate on its use as a methodological tool. Specifically, we hope to show how realism might be used to provide knowledge about the practical implementation of complex healthcare interventions that the current 'gold standard' method of assessment is unable to do. That gold standard is, of course, the randomized control trial (RCT). This involves randomly allocating research subjects into two groups – the intervention group, which receives the intervention, and the control group which does not. Ideally, this allocation should be 'double-blind', whereby neither the researcher nor the research subjects know which group they are in. This is easy in a drug trial where a placebo can look identical to the active medication, but is nigh on impossible in complex interventions which involve changes in the activities of professionals, because at least the professionals involved, if not their clients, will know who is getting what. In either type of RCT, outcomes of both the intervention and control group are measured and statistically analysed to ascertain the degree to which the intervention provides improved health outcomes and the degree to which it leads to negative health consequences. When these are balanced up, the efficacy of the intervention can be ascertained.

This strategy may sound familiar, in that it essentially involves an attempt to approximate the kind of closed system of the classical experiment that we described earlier – the whole aim of randomization and control is to ensure that all things are equal between the two groups with the exception of whether or not the research participants are subjected to the intervention. In other words, we are back to the positivist notion of constant conjunction. In simple terms, if the conjunction of 'take drug, get better' is repeated enough times, while on the other side 'don't take drug, don't get better' is also the predominant conjunction, then we can have reasonable confidence that the drug is efficacious in curing the disease. Leaving aside the problems of specific aetiology discussed above, and accepting that RCTs are a very good way of deciding whether or not drugs work, many healthcare interventions are far more complex in that they involve changing the behaviour of professionals and/or clients. As we have already noted, human behaviour occurs in very open systems with many social, cultural, organizational, psychological and biological factors influencing how we act. We can begin to see how trying to force such complexity into the closed-system binary opposition of 'intervention works/intervention does not work' is going to have its limitations. While it may be possible to artificially construct such a system during the timeframe of an RCT, such closure will break down as soon as the intervention is introduced into everyday practice. This problem was recognized by the great pioneer of RCTs, Archie Cochrane, who observed that 'between the scientific measurements based on RCTs and the benefit measurements...in the community there is a gulf which has been much underestimated' (1972: 2). The problem will also be recognized by anyone who has worked in a clinical setting and wondered why patently good ideas about improvements in care simply peter out or are reduced to empty paper exercises. Reflecting this, the Cochrane Collaboration distinguishes between efficacy – the 'extent to which an intervention produces a beneficial result under ideal conditions' (Green and Higgins 2005: 16) – and effectiveness – the 'extent to which a specific intervention, when used under ordinary circumstances, does what it is intended to do' (2005: 16).

A number of attempts have been made to get around this problem. One concentrates on quantity. Thus, organizations such as the Cochrane Collaboration (Higgins and Green 2008) and the British National Institute for Clinical Excellence (NICE 2006) advocate the use of meta-analyses and systematic reviews as a means of strengthening the information provided by individual trials. The problem here is that more is not really better in that the information still relates exclusively to the characteristics of the intervention and the relationship of constant conjunction between intervention and outcome – other causal mechanisms operating in the open system within which the intervention is implemented remain hidden. Another strategy has been adopted by the Medical Research Council (2000) in the development of a framework for RCTs that evaluate complex interventions, which involves supplementing the RCT with additional phases, aimed at identifying the underlying mechanisms that may influence outcomes prior to the trial and examining the degree to which the intervention can be used effectively in uncontrolled settings after the trial. While this is progress, the RCT remains at the core of the framework, and at the core of the RCT is the assumption that the success or failure of an intervention is determined by its internal characteristics.

Critical realism, with its acceptance of the open nature of the social world in which outcomes are the result of the interaction of a number of causal mechanisms, claims to be able to provide the sort of information that RCTs have signally failed to provide – information that relates to why interventions are effective or ineffective, sustainable or short-lived, in everyday clinical circumstances. The most influential construction of critical realist evaluation is 'realistic evaluation', as developed by Pawson and Tilley (1997). The aim of realistic evaluation is to explain the processes involved between the introduction of an intervention and the outcomes that are produced – in other words, it assumes that the characteristics of the intervention itself are only part of the story, and that the social processes involved in its implementation have to be understood as well if we are going to have an adequate understanding of why observed outcomes come about. In contrast to the assumptions of constant conjunction, realistic evaluation posits the alternative formula of:

$$\text{Mechanism} + \text{context} = \text{outcome}$$

Perhaps it would be better to state mechanisms in the plural, in that in any given context, there will in all likelihood be a number of causal mechanisms in operation, their relationship differing from context to context. The aim of realistic evaluation is to discover if, how and why interventions have the potential to cause beneficial change. To do this, it is necessary to penetrate beneath the surface of observable inputs and outputs in order to uncover how mechanisms which cause problems are removed or countered by alternative mechanisms introduced in the intervention. In turn, this requires an understanding of the contexts within which problem mechanisms operate, and in which intervention mechanisms can be successfully fired. In other words realistic evaluators are once again taking the middle line between positivism and relativism, in that positivism's search for a single cause is seen as too simplistic, while relativism's abandonment of any sort of generalizable explanation is seen as needlessly pessimistic. In contrast to these two poles, realists argue that it is possible to identify tendencies in outcomes (demi-regs in Lawson's terms) that are the result of combinations of causal mechanisms, and to identify the sorts of contexts that will be most auspicious for the success of health-promoting mechanisms. Confidence that the most pertinent tendencies have been identified can be increased through comparison of different cases (i.e., different contexts). In this way, concentration on context – mechanism – outcome configurations allows for the development of transferable and cumulative lessons about the nature of these configurations.

This may all sound well and good, but it is not without its problems, many of which stem from the critical realist strategy of retroduction, which you may remember involves inferring 'from a description of some phenomenon to a description of something which produces it or is a condition for it' (Bhaskar 1986: 11). Two related problems have been succinctly identified by McEvoy and Richards (2003) in their examination of the potential of critical realism as the way forward for evaluation research in nursing:

First, there is the difficulty of finding sufficient grounds to justify assertions that are made about the 'real' existence of causal structures and mechanisms that are invoked to explain natural and social phenomena. Secondly, there is the potential to drift beyond the boundary that separates scientific knowledge from political ideology when making recommendations about the best course of action to follow in any specific set of circumstances. (McEvoy and Richards 2003: 417)

To examine the second objection first, critical realists would argue that the distinction between science and politics is to a degree an artificial one in that our evaluation of interventions should involve an assessment of the degree to which they promote the health, dignity and autonomy of those who are subjected to them; that these human needs should be the criteria by which actions are judged (Doyal and Gough 1991). However, even if we accept that when evaluating human behaviour and its effects on other humans, we cannot be 'value free' and we have to be political with a small 'p', that does not get us over the first objection – how can we be confident that realists are not simply plucking causal mechanisms out of the air? After all, the founder of nursing theory, Florence Nightingale, used realist arguments to demonstrate that causal mechanisms were the laws of an omnipotent God (Porter 2001). While some may agree with such a position, we suspect a great deal more would view this transcendental move of asking the question, 'what must be the case in order for events to occur as they do?' and coming up with the answer of God, as the unsupported and invalid insinuation of Nightingale's metaphysical assumptions into her explanations of health and illness.

It is evident that for critical realism to provide a convincing basis for healthcare evaluation, what is needed is a solidly based foundation of the kind of mechanisms that have been found to operate in healthcare settings. An impressive attempt to provide such a foundation has been developed by Greenhalgh *et al.* (2004), in their systematic review of the literature on the diffusion, dissemination and sustainability of innovations in health service delivery and organization. Essentially, this literature review involved gathering all the evidence available concerning factors involving innovations, organizations and people working in those organizations that have been shown either to promote or to hinder the introduction and sustainability of innovations. They organized this information under nine key headings:

1. The features of the innovation, as perceived by users, decision makers and managers. Here it can be seen that what looks like the traditional evaluation approach which concentrates on the innovation itself is expanded in order to take into account of the fact that it will be viewed differently by different groups of people, which echoes Pawson and Tilley's (1997) description of realistic evaluation as an approach that seeks to uncover what works for whom in what circumstances.
2. The features of the adopters and adoption process.
3. The nature of communication and influence.
4. The organizational context.
5. The state of readiness for a particular innovation.
6. The nature of the wider social and cultural context.
7. The level of planning and resourcing involved.
8. The nature and activities of external agencies.
9. Finally, the outcomes in terms of the rate and extent of adoption or assimilation of the innovation and the extent to which it was sustained and developed.

By systematically reviewing the current literature, Greenhalgh *et al.*'s review provides a flexible template for assessing the implementation of healthcare interventions in that it allows an evaluator to empirically examine the implementation of a particular intervention in a particular context in terms of all the areas listed above. It then facilitates the researcher to make a grounded assessment of its success or otherwise, along with reasons why, on the basis of comparing the context that they have examined with past precedents as outlined in the review of previous cases cited in Greenhalgh *et al.*'s literature review.

While providing a platform for evaluation that allows us to take account of the complexity of the introduction of interventions, the degree to which Greenhalgh *et al.*'s model can be described as critical realism is not entirely clear, in that it is difficult to decipher what constitutes a mechanism, or what is merely a description of a surface characteristic of a particular organization or actor. While Greenhalgh *et al.* commend the use of realistic evaluation, their model does not confine itself narrowly to critical realist philosophy or methodology. Nevertheless, leaving issues of philosophical orthodoxy to one side, their model provides a potentially invaluable route for healthcare researchers who recognize the shortcomings of traditional evaluation approaches and who wish to assess interventions in terms of process instead of just looking at the characteristics of the interventions themselves. The model also has the benefit of being constructed in such a way as to promote interdisciplinary and mixed methods research, thus encouraging researchers to come out of their occupational and methodological bunkers.

At the moment, the jury is still out as to whether critical realist approaches have the capacity to fill the gap that traditional approaches have been unable to fill. While numerous projects are underway, completed studies are not numerous. One example can be found in Byng *et al.*'s (2005) realistic evaluation of practice-level interventions with people with long-term mental illness. Similarly, Kazi (2003a, 2003b) has used critical realism to evaluate social work practice. While ground-breaking and informative, all of these studies provide not a little evidence of the difficulty for researchers in translating high theory into practical evaluation. However, it is early days yet, with an increasing number of studies using this approach in the pipeline. Only time will tell the degree to which critical realism can provide a successful approach to understanding healthcare.

Conclusion and new directions for healthcare

In this chapter, we hope that we have managed to map out how critical realism positions itself as an alternative to the two traditional
poles of social theory. On the one hand, it rejects the structuralist
notion of individual behaviour being determined by society, and the
positivist notion that behaviour can be explained by uncovering laws
of cause and effect. On the other hand, it equally rejects the view that
everything can be reduced to the individual level, or that, because of
the uniqueness of individuals and individual settings, it is impossible
to generate generalized knowledge about society. Instead, it posits the
existence of causal mechanisms that influence and pattern people's
behaviour, but which interact with each other in differing ways in
different circumstances, so that their power involves generating tendencies, rather than constant conjunctions. For critical realists, while
people are not automatons governed by social laws, they are nevertheless resourced and constrained by the structured relationships
within which they find themselves.

Moving from a general theoretical position, we hope that from the
chosen examples, you have got a flavour of how critical realism
aspires to provide a fuller understanding of the causes of health and
illness. In the first example, the critique of specific aetiology, realism
argued that there was a need to broaden causative explanations in
that illness could rarely be explained by recourse to a simple cause
and effect relationship with a single factor, be that factor a germ or a
gene. Instead, the relationship of a number of causative factors, that
would take different forms in different circumstances, needed to be
taken into account. Similarly, in relation to the disability debate, the
critical realist position argues that seeing disability as exclusively
the result of bodily impairment or social oppression provides too narrow a basis for understanding the complex relationship between body
and society. In the example of inequalities in health, critical realism
involved observing the need for deeper causative explanations than
those currently being offered. While observations that poverty and
inequality are associated with inequalities in health are significant
findings, they are not sufficient, in that they cannot explain why
social inequalities are so stark, and getting starker. In order to find
that out, there is a need to uncover the causative mechanisms generated by structured economic relations.

In our look at how critical realism might contribute to understandings of healthcare, we adopted a more technical approach, showing

how supporters of realistic evaluation claim that it can gain knowledge about the processes that contribute to the success or failure of health-care innovations that other approaches to evaluation are unable to uncover. Once again, their argument is based around the critical realist critique of both positivism and relativism.

So what about future directions in research? Starting with the last first, there is much activity going on in health services research involving empirical researchers who have recognized the shortcomings of current strategies to explain why interventions work or do not work in practical settings, irrespective of their demonstrated efficacy. Critical realism, and in particular realistic evaluation, promises a route out of this extremely frustrating impasse, and that promise is currently being tested through practical research. The results of that research over the next few years will see whether the promise can be fulfilled.

Moving back another step in the chapter to the problem of inequalities in health, we would argue that, given the almost universal drift in the Western world towards increased inequality in both income and health, it is only a matter of time before the concerns of critical realists and Marxists return to the forefront of research and, indeed, popular discourse. As the problem becomes starker, so it becomes less easy to avoid the 'why' question: why is this seemingly inexorable drift away from common human experience happening? What are the fundamentals that are causing it? While these questions have been successfully evaded during the long boom in which more people have become better off and live longer, albeit at vastly differential rates, the end to that boom will leave a lot of people demanding explanations, which will hopefully prompt a more critical attitude from those who make a living out of explaining health and illness and their causations. Or maybe not.

Critical realism's intervention in the disability debate involves the attempt to steer away from exclusively social or biological reductions and the associated division of disability into separate spheres of bio-medicine and social activism. Whether or not disability activists will find this line progressive in that it opens up biomedicine's monopoly over the conception and treatment of physical impairment to debate and challenge, or, conversely, whether it will be viewed as a Trojan horse that entails the covert reintroduction of the old fixation on impairment to the detriment of efforts to achieve the social emancipation of those labelled as disabled, it is too early to tell.

Finally, the genetic question: once again, it is not that difficult to make the argument that critical realism provides a more comprehensive and calibrated explanation than rival models because it does not make unconvincing reductions that adopt either nature or nurture as their exclusive mantra. It would therefore be reasonable to assume that realism has the potential to provide a framework for future, balanced research. But perhaps this assumption is the epitome of idealism in that the slow and measured steps of rigorous research often provide a poor challenge to the quick and easy answers of unmeasured journalism. This is a battle of ideas that will be well worth watching.

CHAPTER 6

Feminist Theory, Health and Healthcare

Introduction

In this chapter, we identify the central principles of feminist theory and consider their application to our understanding of both health and healthcare. Like many perspectives, feminist theory is a broad church and is cross-cut by a range of other approaches to social theory. In exploring feminist theory, we outline various shifts, overlaps and tensions that have emerged within feminist thinking over the past five decades. A central perspective within feminist theory, upon which we will expand, is the concept of gender. Gender is perceived to be socially produced, and as Widerberg (2000) notes, each historical epoch creates its own meaning regarding gender that mediates the structure and social processes of a particular society. However, the extent to which biological differences between the sexes can be written out of the picture has been a matter for debate within feminist theory, an issue that we consider in relation to the principles of feminist theory.

The attempt to unpack the principles of feminist theory is followed by an exploration of how feminist theory contributes to our understanding of health. Here, we consider the gendered patterning of health and illness in terms of mortality, morbidity and the diagnosis and treatment of disease; the way in which gender mediates how health, illness and bodies are socially constructed; and the manner in which women make sense of health and illness from their own perspectives. Finally we turn to applications of feminist theory to understandings of healthcare. In this section, we consider the application of feminist theory to our understanding of healthcare in relation to three interrelated issues: the gendered social organization of healthcare; gender issues in healthcare interactions; and the women's health movement. In the conclusion, we consider new directions for research and return to the enduring question of the place of biology in relation to gender in future health research.

Principles of feminist theory

Feminist theory is a woman-centred area of scholarship aimed at understanding and analysing the position and status of women in society. Humm proposes that:

> Feminist theory is fundamentally about women's experience. Its subject is women's past and contemporary history and through utilising, and often rejecting, the explanations of economics, religion, or politics it brings into consciousness undiscovered aspects of women's lives. (Humm 1995: xiii)

Madoo Lengermann and Niebrugge-Brantley (2003) assert that the woman-centredness of feminist theory is manifested in three ways. First, the central focus or 'objects' of enquiry are the experiences and context of women's lives. Second, women themselves are the key 'subjects' in the research process from whose perspective knowledge about the world is produced (a perspective known as the feminist standpoint position) (Smith 1988). Third, feminist theory has a political goal in activating for social transformation on women's behalf for the betterment of humankind, that is, the empowerment of women. In this regard, it shares a commitment to social reform with critical social theory. The empowerment of women is concerned with challenging patriarchy – the domination of women by men. First introduced by Max Weber ([1922] 1978) to refer to the domination of family members by the eldest male, patriarchy is used by feminist writers both to describe the social position of women and as a means of theorizing their social position (Best 2003).

Gender – a central concept within feminist theory as indicated earlier – is defined by Kegan Gardiner (2005: 35) as '...the idea that masculinity and femininity are loosely defined, historically variable, and interrelated social ascriptions to persons with certain kinds of bodies – not the natural, necessary, or ideal characteristics of people with similar genitals'. Indeed, she posits that the identification of gender as a social construction is the most significant achievement of twentieth-century feminist theory. The definition advanced by Wharton, drawing on Ridgeway and Smith-Lovin (1999: 192), illuminates the concept further, whereupon gender is defined as a:

> system of social practices [that] creates and maintains gender distinctions and [...] organises relations of inequality on the basis of [these distinctions]. In this view, gender involves the creation of both differences and inequalities. (Wharton 2005: 7)

But what of biological differences between the sexes, and how far they might go in explaining the different experiences of men and women? As Fausto-Sterling (2003: 124) notes, if there is an identifiable component of 'naked sex' from which gender can be disentangled, the question remains as to how much this accounts for gender difference. We will consider this burning issue for feminist theory as we trace its developments.

Feminist theory emerged within academic feminism predominantly since the 1970s in the West in a climate of second-wave[1] feminism, although there were political theses advocating political and social equality for women long before this (Evans 2003) (e.g., Mary Astell's *A Serious Proposal to the Ladies* was published in 1694 and Mary Wollstonecraft's *Vindication of the Rights of Women* in 1792). Widerberg (2000: 469) delineates three phases in contemporary feminist research in which different aspects dominated: the phase of theory critique; the phase of making visible or 'visiblising'; and the phase of reflectivity. The first phase involved a critique of classical social theory, and in particular the notion of value-neutrality and objective knowledge associated with positivism. A feminist reading of classical sociological scholarship also drew attention to the primacy of the masculine subject in accounts of the emergence of modern society (Adkins 2005). For example, central issues in the classical texts were the events of rapid urbanization, the

---

[1] Second-wave feminism denotes a period of feminist activity that started towards the end of the 1960s, and endured until the late 1970s. While first-wave feminism was concerned with transforming legal barriers to equality for women, second-wave feminism exposed unofficial inequalities also.

political consciousness of wage labour (see the discussion on Marx in Chapter 2), or the condition of alienation or anomie (see the discussion on Durkheim in Chapter 1); these, feminists argued, were more closely aligned with explaining social change from the perspective of men rather than women (Adkins 2005). Although Weber proposed that traditional modes of power involved partriarchal domination (rule by the father and husband), as Adkins (2005: 235) notes, women's dependency was understood as a consequence of the 'normal superiority of the physical and intellectual energies of the male'. During this phase of theory critique, the concepts of power and interest in the production of knowledge also became central, leading to a 'new' women's movement in the universities, with women organizing on their own to critique theoretical perspectives (Widerberg 2000).

The phase of visibilizing represented a shift in focus from critiquing theory to constructing concepts and theories from the perspectives of women's lived experiences (a feminist standpoint position). In this sense, women's situations would be examined on their own terms, without reference to those of men. The third phase, that of reflectivity, arising out of the empirical work of the preceding phase, involved a questioning attitude to the research produced in the visiblizing phase. In addition, the reflectivity phase involved the beginning of a shift towards the deconstruction of 'woman' as an analytical category. This last phase paralleled poststructuralist thinking (see Chapter 4), although as Widerberg (2000: 477) observes, 'the women researchers continued to keep one foot outside this paradigm'. In particular, the notion of focusing solely on women's experiences in attempting to understand gender became a focus of critical debate; the view that all knowledge is socially produced meant that the authenticity of both feminists and women's discursively constructed accounts also became questionable (Davis 2007).

Within the academy, with which second-wave feminism has engaged (Evans 2003: 8), the 1990s saw the term 'gender studies' superseding the term 'women's studies' for both political and intellectual reasons. While the central focus of the academic work continued to be gender difference, the shift represented an acknowledgement that the manner in which gender was constructed involved men as well as women (Evans 2003). A new and parallel field of study, Critical Studies on Men and Masculinities (CSM) has grown up, concerned with exploring and theorizing the gendered construction of men's lives, generally without seeking to re-exclude women. Men's movements more broadly have varied in terms of their relationship to feminism.

Kegan Gardiner (2005: 47) observes that while masculinist movements at times discredit feminism, 'generally men's studies treat feminism and feminist theory as scholarly big sisters, perhaps dull, dowdy, outmoded, or too restrictive, but nevertheless models to be followed and bettered'.

Evans (1995) identifies as a central issue in feminist theory the extent to which women are believed to be similar or dissimilar from men. This she coins the 'equality-difference controversy' (Evans 1995: 3), or as some would put it, the sameness-difference debate. Sameness feminists, she proposes, demand equal treatment for men and women, for example, in recruitment to and entitlements in employment. Evans (1995: 13) argues that second-wave feminism of the 1960s represented two types of 'equality' (or sameness) schools, namely, liberal feminism and what she labels 'early radical' feminism. Liberal feminism proposed that there were no differences between men and women that justified discrimination on the basis of sex. Any differences that manifested themselves other than the most basic biological differences were theorized as being the product of socialization, or of medical or mass media discourses and so forth. As Evans notes,

> Liberal equality feminism [...] asks for equality in the sense of sameness of attainment, and therefore treatment, and justifies it via sameness, androgyny. It says: we deserve to be equal with you, for we are in fact the same. We possess the same capabilities; but this fact has been hidden, or these abilities have, while still potentially ours, been socialized, educated, 'out'. (Evans 1995: 13)

Evans refers to such liberal feminist thinkers as 'sameness' thinkers who attempt to demonstrate the paucity of psychological, behavioural and linguistic differences between men and women.

Theorists such as Shulamith Firestone (1971) from the early radicalism school, the second of the equality perspectives delineated by Evans, held that patriarchy impacted negatively on both men and women in sustaining a system of hierarchy, subjugation and exploitation. What distinguishes radical feminism is its contention that all types of oppression are rooted in male supremacy (Humm 1995). As Evans (1995: 63) notes, 'In major and more fully fledged theory, the roots of all oppression were argued to lie in the oppression of women – and sometimes children – so that with their liberation, with the gaining of equality for them, would come freedom and equality for all humankind.' Early radicalism had no shared perspective on how exactly a revised society might be socially organized or brought about (Evans 1995). Although it denounces all forms of oppression, rank and hierarchy, radical feminism focuses on sexuality as a site of patriarchy (Evans 1995). Sex is perceived to be a key to women's oppression (Best 2003), most specifically in the manner in which sex is ideologically constructed around the penis (Thompson 2001). The radical perspective holds that in patriarchal society women accept their inferior status and subordinate themselves to men's sexual desire. Heterosexuality is not viewed as an individual choice that people subscribe to, or fixed by psychological childhood processes, but rather as a socially constructed arrangement (Millett 1977), with heterosexuality imposed upon women through social regulation (Rich 1977). All acts of heterosexual sex are interpreted as a manifestation of male power. Thus, for radical feminists such as Denise Thompson (2001), masculinity is the root of all forms of subordination.

Within this sameness-difference debate, just how the female body should be interpreted has been a central tension. For sameness theorists, the achievement of equality becomes possible only by transcending the female body (Davis 2007) since claims that women's bodies and bodily experiences are different to those of men run the risk of falling back into old essentialist arguments, that is, that there are essential biological differences between men and women that determine their experiences and behaviour. The concern for sameness theorists is that biological determinism might then continue to be used to justify different expectations and rules of conduct for males and females that feminism attempts to overcome. Difference feminists, by contrast, reject the notion that the female body should be transcended for the purposes of equality and instead have canvassed for affirming the uniqueness of the female body, for example, in its capacity to bear and breastfeed children (Davis 2007). They favour drawing attention to the physical and experiential differences between men and women that have their roots in the body (Howson 2005). The notion of embodiment – the perceptual experience of the body's engagement with the world – has been a central theoretical perspective within difference feminism. It is closely linked with phenomenology, discussed in Chapter 3, and the view that consciousness may only be understood through the lived experience of the body.

Difference feminists also argue that society is socially organized around men's needs, and this organization becomes seen as normal

(Evans 1995). Any demands that women make to modify this 'normal' arrangement, ostensibly catering for 'people' but in effect designed to meet men's needs, are viewed as special requests. This male-orientated society thus fails to be problematized, mitigating against the establishment of a new social order that accommodates and legitimates at its core the needs of both men and women. Thus difference theorists do not want women to fit in to an existing masculinist social arrangement, but rather want to transform that social arrangement to fully and legitimately accommodate the needs of women (see Evans 1995).

Not all feminist thought can be clearly positioned within either the equality or difference perspectives, and, owing to historical shifts in thinking, socialist feminism is one such example. Traditionally, socialist feminism was distinguished by the centrality it afforded to the link between patriarchy and capitalism in explaining women's oppression. The view is that women are particularly exploited within capitalism and that the roots of women's oppression lie in the total economic mode of production of capitalism, encompassing not just women's relationship to the means of production, but also their social experience of that economic system. Ehrenreich (1976) proposes that the historical context of capitalism is crucial to any attempt to understand sexism as it is played out in everyday contexts. One of the aspirations of socialist feminism, Ehrenreich writes, is:

> to transform not only the ownership of the means of production, but the totality of social existence. [...] Because we see monopoly capitalism as a political/economic/cultural totality, we have room within our Marxist framework for feminist issues which have nothing ostensibly to do with production or 'politics', issues that have nothing to do with family, health care, 'private' life. (Ehrenreich 1976: 4)

Ehrenreich proposes that the factors that have 'atomized' working-class life and that underpin a cultural and material dependency on the bourgeoisie are exactly those that maintain the subjugation of women. Thus, socialist feminists highlight the linkages between women's struggles and class struggle. However, Evans (1995) notes that socialist feminism has shifted over time in relation to the concept of equality it holds. In recent years the aspiration of achieving radical equality though 'sameness equality' has been superseded by an emphasis on sex and gender difference.

Madoo Lengermann and Niebrugge-Brantley (2003: 443) argue that theories of gender difference must account for what is coined 'the essentialist argument' – the notion that there are identifiable differences between men and women, associated with three factors: (i) biological differences; (ii) different social institutional needs to enable men and women to fulfil different roles, particularly linked to the family; and (iii) the peripheral status of women as 'Other' in a male-produced culture.

With regard to the first of these – biological differences – feminist scholars (with notable exceptions such as Alice Rossi (1977, 1983) have tended to favour cultural explanations for accounting for the way in which men and women are different. This way of thinking is generally referred to as cultural feminism, and focuses on the different values that women have compared with men in their ways of being. Such theoretical accounts have drawn attention to positive female characteristics such as women's capacity to be caring, their non-violent approach to resolving conflict, lower levels of aggression and their ability to communicate emotional experiences, which suggest that women have different standards for ethical judgements (see Madoo Lengermann and Niebrugge-Brantley 2003). This contrasts with a traditionally masculine type of ethical reasoning based on the principles of rationality, impartiality, justice and objectivity. This field of feminist theory contributes to a discourse on caring referred to as the feminist ethic of care, which balances reason with context and permits emotional engagement in ethical decision-making (Gilligan 1982, see also Noddings 1984, and Sherwin 1992). These notions are played out in feminist research methodologies which critique conventional research conduct for failing to develop a knowledge based on women's experiences and for overlooking the pervasive effects of gender on the research process (Oakley 1981, Finch 1984, Graham 1984, Letherby 2003); these ideas also permeate much feminist theory. In a general sense, cultural feminism proposes that women's ways of being and knowing are different from those of men, and may herald a better, more just society than the established cultural practices designed by and primarily for men.

In relation to the second notion – that women have different social institutional needs to those of men – the perspective here is that gender differences arise from the diverse roles that men and women occupy within institutional contexts (Madoo Lengermann and Niebrugge-Brantley 2003). Women's historical position in the domestic sphere, for example, gives rise to a particular set of experiences and relational positions, especially concerning the division of labour that links them to the role of wife and mother. The third theme above regarding women's marginal status refers to the way in which women have been relegated as 'Other' in a male-constructed culture as revealed in Simone de Beauvoir's classic work *The Second Sex* ([1949/1957] 1989), and by numerous feminist writers since (see Madoo Lengermann and Niebrugge-Brantley). Within this male-centred culture, there is an assumption of male as subject from whose vantage point the world is constructed and defined. Women's experiences and conceptual framing of the world are marginalized, and at its most extreme, woman is constructed as 'the Other' – 'an objectified being who is assigned traits that represent the opposite of the agentic, subject male' (Madoo Lengermann and Niebrugge-Brantley 2003: 445).

A more recent current in feminist theory, feminist postmodernism is rooted in a rejection of universalism, and celebrates the demise of all definitive proclamations of truth. Postmodernist ideas began to permeate feminist thinking in the 1990s. Feminist postmodernists advance the notion of plurality in knowledge development and reject the kind of essentialism promoted by cultural feminism. They challenge the notion that there is something 'unique' or authoritative about women's experiences, instead proposing that these are an outcome of cultural discourses, that is, they are socially constructed through language, material organization and institutional practices, and are thus variable. Evans (1995: 125) observes that some people associate feminist postmodernism with acknowledging differences between individual women, but she interprets it as a theory that emphasizes 'a "difference within", the fragmentation of the self'. Unlike radical or socialist feminists who assume that the category 'woman' is unambiguous, and liberal feminists who argue for equal treatment for men and women, postmodernist feminists deconstruct the category 'woman'. In the work of writers such as Judith Butler (1990), the notion that women have a shared identity is problematized, with the emphasis instead on the way in which gender mediates other dimensions of identity. It is through language, according to Butler, that gender identities are constructed and constituted. Thus, the assumption that there is an *a priori* 'truth' about sex that constitutes the gendered person is challenged. Gender identity is not deemed to precede language; instead, gender is something that we perform and something that we accept as a 'reality', a perspective that is developed through the notion of 'performativity' (Butler 1990). Butler's work and that of other postmodern feminist theorists has been criticized for its lack of attention to the material reality of the body (Kuhlmann and Babitsch 2002, Davis 2007). The concern here is that while the body has become the central theoretical focus by deconstructing dualisms and biological essentialism, the material aspects of the body are theorized away, hence ignoring the embodied dimensions of people's lives (how we come to occupy and experience our physical bodies).

Fraser and Nicholson (1988) explore the manner in which 'metanarratives' (ideas intended to offer an overarching explanation of experience or knowledge) that traditionally underpinned social analysis have begun to lose their credibility, and generalizations inherent in assumptions about women across all cultures have begun to dissipate. However, they do not propose that all meta-narratives be abandoned, but rather that the focus of postmodernist feminist theory would be comparative instead of universalizing. McLennan (1995) observes a hesitancy in postmodernist feminist work such as that of Hekman (1990), Nicholson (1990, 1992), and Flax (1990) to gravitate towards a strong postmodernist position, because of the danger that feminism as a distinctive theory and practice might be demolished through theoretical pluralism. Writers such as Holmwood (1995) suggest that the competing and mutually exclusive epistemological positions within feminist theory constitute a crisis on a par with that in mainstream social theory.

A parallel feminist movement is Black feminist thought, or Afrocentric feminist thought. It has been defined by Hill Collins as consisting of:

> specialized knowledge created by African-American women which clarifies a standpoint of and for Black women. In other words, Black feminist thought encompasses theoretical interpretations of Black women's reality by those who live it. (Hill Collins 2001: 155)

This perspective embraces class, race and gender as interconnected systems of oppression (Hill Collins 2001), and refutes 'additive approaches' to oppression. By additive approaches is meant the notion of beginning with gender and then adding social divides such as class, age, sexual orientation, race and religion. Black feminist thought, by contrast, views these sites of oppressions as interlocking components of one overarching system of domination.

While our account presented here indicates that feminist theory has both influenced and been influenced by historical developments in social theory, Adkins (2005: 233–234) argues that it is misleading to interpret the history of feminist theory in terms of a simple shift from Enlightenment thinking encompassing universalist values of rationality, reason and equality to 'post-Enlightenment' values concerned with 'difference', 'specificity' and 'particularism'. She asserts that assuming this trajectory in the roll-out of feminist theory does not account for the way that the category of gender is being re-conceptualized by contemporary feminist theorists, in full acknowledgement of the shortcomings of Enlightenment thinking. Hemmings (2005) argues a similar case, in which she challenges dominant narratives about how Western second-wave feminist theory has developed. She argues that dominant perspectives have become fixed within particular decades, with one approach being presented as displacing another or set against one another. She advocates emphasizing the continuities rather than the fissures in feminist theory developments.

Applications to understandings of health

In recent years, there has been a plethora of research papers highlighting the way in which gender mediates the patterning of health and illness, how it impacts upon the way in which health and illness come to be defined, and how it cross-cuts the experience of health and illness. As is the case with other theoretical positions presented in this book, researchers focusing on gender issues in health do not tend to explicitly align themselves with one particular theoretical paradigm in making sense of their data, but are rather inclined to invoke a position that might generally span a number of overlapping theoretical perspectives. Thus, it is not an easy task to present perspectives on health and illness that identify easily with, for example, the kind of feminisms outlined in the previous section, such as a liberal feminist or a socialist feminist position. Nonetheless, we can trace shifts in research on the topic of gender and health to developments in feminist thinking and indeed identify general themes in research on health and illness that are informed by a feminist perspective. These themes, which we expand upon forthwith, are the following:

- The gendered patterning of mortality and morbidity.
- The way in which gender mediates how health, illness and bodies are socially constructed.
- How women make sense of health and illness from their own perspectives.

The gendered patterning of mortality and morbidity

Feminist theorists have been concerned with differences in the health status of men and women emerging from research. If we examine work in this area, we can link some of the developments in historical thinking within feminism outlined in the first section on feminist theory with shifts in scholarship on the gendered patterning of health. If we begin in the 1970s when gender entered the agenda of health studies, we see that the notion of women's health was treated as an undifferentiated category, and a conventional wisdom emerged that whilst women tended to live longer than men, they suffered from poorer health. This excess in morbidity experienced by women was explained through the notion of gender (rather than biology), namely, that women's structural disadvantage and family roles were largely responsible for the disparity between the sexes.

What emerged in the 1990s was a challenge to the conventional wisdom that women consistently fared worse than men in terms of morbidity (Macintyre *et al.* [1996] 2004, Mathews *et al.* 1999); rather, more fine-grain analyses of how morbidity is cross-cut by 'time, place, specific health conditions and age' gave rise to the notion that women do not consistently suffer from poorer health compared with men (Hunt and Annandale 1999: 1). Furthermore, the concept of gender began to be broadened out to encompass and address the circumstances of men as well as those of women, mirroring developments more generally within feminist scholarship (e.g., Hunt and Annandale (1999), referring to a special edition of *Social Science and Medicine* that they edited in 1999, indicated that all but one of the papers on gender and morbidity concerned the health of both men and women). Research on men's health has consistently focused on men's poorer health in relation to the major causes of death and lower life expectancy in Western societies and draws a link between a pattern of men's poor health behaviours (such as adoption of high health risk activities and a reluctance to seek general health and medical advice) and hegemonic cultural constructs of masculinities, frequently defined in terms of male stoicism and masculine invincibility (Lohan 2007: 498). Courtnenay's (2000) analysis, focusing on the higher mortality rate for men and their poor standing in relation to some severe chronic conditions, emphasizes the *beliefs* and *behaviours* of men that undermine their health. The author notes that these beliefs and behaviours are characteristics of hegemonic masculinity and are invoked by men to negotiate status and power: the closer that men identify with hegemonic masculinity by taking risks in relation to their health the more 'men legitimize themselves as the stronger sex' (Courtnenay 2000: 1397).

Lohan (2007: 498) has noted that, on the one hand, studies of men's health need to be able to acknowledge, where necessary, the relative stability of cultural notions of masculinity on men's health. On the other hand, they need to also take on board the poststructuralist feminist concern to avoid essentializing characteristics, such as risk adversity, aggression and competitiveness as 'masculine' or endemic in masculine culture. She goes on to note that a key mechanism within Critical Studies on Men for taking culture seriously but avoiding cultural reductionism is prioritizing a research focus on diversity in how masculinity and health operate in daily lives between men. In addition, cultural reductionism may also be circumvented by highlighting how individual men do not approach all health practices in a consistent way, and moreover, their health perspectives and practices are cross-cut by social divides such as ethnicity, sexual orientation and socio-economic status (see, e.g., O'Brien *et al.* 2005, Robertson 2006a, Oliffe 2008).

Similarly reflecting developments within feminist theory, research papers on the gendered patterning of health from the 1990s onwards began to focus on disparities among women themselves that arise by virtue of social divides such class (Chen *et al.* 2005), ethnicity (Bell *et al.* 2006, Dabral Datta *et al.* 2006, Grann *et al.* 2006) and changing roles and responsibilities (Wickrama *et al.* 2006). Thus, it was no longer a case of merely highlighting the health status of women *vis-à-vis* men, but rather of elucidating diversity among women as a differentiated category at various stages of the life course (see, e.g., studies by Boneham and Sixsmith 2006, Cwikel *et al.* 2006, McMunn *et al.* 2006). In spite of shifts in feminist theory influencing the field of health research over the years, the notion that gender, that is, socially constructed roles and relations between the sexes, influences patterns of mortality and morbidity has been an enduring theme (Arber and Khlat 2002).

The way in which gender mediates how health, illness and bodies are socially constructed

Some feminist theorists have attempted to explain health and illness by focusing on how the patriarchal medical establishment has medicalized aspects of female behaviour and social practices and turned them into pathologies or potential pathologies in order to control the female body. Let us pause to look at the concept of medicalization. The term 'medicalization' was first introduced by Irving Zola (1972), who applied it to a number of issues, namely: the expansion of areas deemed to be relevant to medicine; the retention by medicine of absolute control over specific technical procedures; medicine's privileged access to taboo areas; and the expansion of what in medicine is considered to be relevant to healthy living. The term is generally used to refer to the tendency for everyday events and social problems to be defined in medical terms, with the labels 'healthy' and 'ill' being viewed as relevant to a greater number of activities of living.[2] As noted in Chapter 2, medicalization is also seen as a cause and consequence of the professional dominance of medicine in healthcare (Freidson 1970b). Feminists critical of the medicalization of women's bodies argue that medicine is not merely dealing with objective categories of diseases that 'exist' within the human body and arise because of aberrations in bodily functions, but rather creates or socially constructs types of illness whereupon the social realm (e.g., gender) cross-cuts the physical dimension to give rise to a medical diagnosis or a type of disorder. In this way, societal values, expectations and norms about gender may influence the diagnosis and treatment of a disease or disorder, or even whether a state of affairs comes to be considered a disease or disorder in the first place.

A strong theme of feminist work in this area is to resist the medicalization of women's bodies, that is, the way in which everyday aspects of life such as pregnancy, birth, menopause, ageing and so on have come under the jurisdiction of medicine. For example, much feminist writing has centred on the way in which women's reproductive anatomy, physiology and hormones have been defined as pathological or potentially pathological within medical discourses. Feminist writers have linked the historical oppression of women to how women's bodies and minds were constructed within medical discourses – as being irrational, emotional and ruled by their hormones (see Lupton 2003). This gendered way of viewing the female body influenced the perception that women were fit for certain types of work and not others, and

---

[2] Conrad (1992, Conrad and Schneider 1992, Conrad and Angell 2004) has also developed the concept of medicalization pointing to the shift from religious to medical control of behaviours in contemporary 'secular' societies. In addition, recent work by Conrad and colleagues examines how a new range of conditions such as andropause and baldness (Szymczak and Conrad 2006) and ADHD (Conrad and Potter 2000) have been brought under the rubric of medicine.

impacted on the positions that they were allowed or encouraged to occupy in society. As Lorber puts it:

> despite the strong evidence of women's overall physical hardiness, *all* [emphasis in the original] women are considered unfit for certain kinds of work and physical activity because of their procreative physiology. What supposedly makes females 'real' women – their menstrual cycles – makes them unreliable workers, thinkers, and leaders. (Lorber 1997: 55)

Similarly, the construction of pregnancies and birth as potentially risky medicalizes these life events, locating all pregnant and birthing women under medical control (Murphy-Lawless 1998; for an analysis of the gendered medicalization of men's bodies, see Rosenfeld and Faircloth 2006).

In the earlier section on feminist theory, we referred to de Beauvoir's ([1949/1957] 1989) critique of the way in which society centralizes the male subject from whose vantage point the world is defined, while the female subject is relegated as Other; this perspective is invoked by a number of feminist writers and historians in relation to how the female body was perceived prior to the nineteenth century within medical discourses. Such scholars have criticized what they interpret to be a 'one-sex' male-centric model of viewing the body that gave primacy to the male body as the norm against which the female body could be judged (see Ehrenreich and English 1974, Schiebinger 1989, 2003a, Laqueur 1990). While this conceptualization has been challenged by medical historians (Churchill 2005), a more recent analysis of anatomy textbooks for medical students in the United States noted that in illustrations, vocabulary and syntax, these texts portrayed the male anatomy as the norm to which female anatomical features were compared; the 'human body' was primarily manifested as the male body (Lawrence and Bendixen 1992).

Mental illness is another realm that has interested feminist theorists who argue that within the discipline of psychiatry, gendered versions of health, illness and therapies are constructed and reproduced. Chesler (1972) highlighted how categories of masculinity and femininity were generated within the discipline of psychiatry; female behaviour such as lesbianism was pathologized, and passivity deemed normal for women. More recent studies of psychiatry have found that normative perspectives on gender are reproduced and reinforced in the therapeutic relationship in the treatment of eating disorders (Moulding 2006). Moulding (2006: 802–803) noted that although a rhetoric of choice and autonomy were associated with treatment programmes, the actual narratives of health practitioners concerning bed rest and psychotherapy smacked of 'a gendered parental dynamic that ultimately seeks to control women and girls and ironically reproduces the negative and controlling family dynamics commonly theorized within psycho-medicine as typical of the "anorexic family"'.

Other gender-focused scholarship has drawn attention to the gender-typing of particular conditions. A case in point is the depiction of migraine as demonstrated in Kempner's (2006: 1986) analysis of the marketing practices of pharmaceutical companies, whereupon migraine is presented as a 'woman's disorder'. Further evidence of gender-typing is presented in a semiotic analysis of marketing data in which depression was found to be constructed as a female disease and cardiovascular disease a male disease (Curry and O'Brien 2006). Curry and O'Brien's (2006) research indicated that medical publications' advertisings for cardiovascular and antidepressant drugs reproduce gender stereotypes by portraying men as the main consumers of cardiovascular drugs, and women the primary users of antidepressant medication. They argue that although younger men are more at risk of suicide, they were never portrayed in the antidepressant drug advertisements studied. Rather, advertisements for anti-depressants presented depression as natural for females, while those for cardiovascular drugs tended to show men engaged in physical activities and rarely in the 'sick role'. Constructing masculinity and femininity in this way may influence men to deny experiences of depression, associating it with powerlessness and a lack of autonomy (Curry and O'Brien 2006). Presenting cardiovascular disease as a male disease misrepresents the evidence that cardiovascular disease was the cause of 39 per cent of female deaths in the United States for the year 2003 (American Heart Association 2007). It has been argued that the gender stereotyping of particular conditions may lead to medical professionals under-diagnosing them, and concomitantly inhibiting therapeutic interventions (Curry and O'Brien 2006, Kempner 2006). Indeed, there is evidence that this occurs – women with comparable symptoms to men have been found to be less likely to receive cardiac diagnostic tests and interventions (Steingart *et al.* 1991, Di Cecco *et al.* 2002, Burnstein *et al.* 2003).

The gendering of particular conditions has been found to occur even at the stage of clinical trials for particular treatments. Schiebinger (2003b) cites several major US studies relating to cardiovascular disease that excluded women, predominantly because the menstrual cycle is perceived to be a methodological complication that increases the cost of the research. She argues that the exclusion of women in this way puts them at risk of adverse drug reactions; such adverse reactions arise twice as often with women than men. The situation in terms of inclusion in medical research improved greatly for women from the late 1980s with the instigation of the Office of Research on Women's Health in the United States at national level (Schiebinger 2003b).

How women make sense of health and illness from their own perspectives

Following trends in feminist theory towards visiblizing the world from the perspective of women themselves, a plethora of studies on women's experiences of various health issues has emerged, predominantly since the 1990s. Much of the critique of women's absence from health research was cross-cut by a criticism of the established methodologies – predominantly quantitative – that were deemed to silence women and reduce their experiences to quantifiable units of analysis (Graham 1983). Thus, studies since this period focusing on women's health experiences tend to employ qualitative methodologies that aim to centralize the experiences of women. The emphasis in this canon of studies is highly varied, and includes phenomenological research that focuses on women's bodies and embodied experiences (Dalsgaard Reventlow *et al.* 2006), living with a serious or chronic condition (Doyal and Anderson 2005, Manderson *et al.* 2005, Martínez 2005, Press *et al.* 2005, Takahashi and Kai 2005), and women's experiences of pregnancy and childbirth (El-Nemer *et al.* 2006, Fisher *et al.* 2006, Kendall *et al.* 2005, Liamputtong 2005, Williams *et al.* 2005). Emily Martin (2001) adopted both a phenomenological and a structural critique of women's social position along with a discourse analysis of cultural metaphors about women's bodies to understand their embodied experiences of menstruation and menopause. We also see a genre of work emerging on Black women's experiences of illness that theorize data in relation to ethnicity (see, e.g., Doyal and Anderson 2005, Edge and Rogers 2005), reflecting the shift in feminist thinking to acknowledging diversity in experiences and a deconstruction of the unitary concept of 'woman'. It is also worth bearing in mind that health research on women does not necessarily equate with feminist health research; the latter tends to be distinguished by the explicitness of its political purpose.

As indicated in the earlier section on feminist theory, we noted the development of the field of study, Critical Studies on Men and Masculinities aimed at theorizing how men's lives are gendered. We see this trend in a broadening out of the health research agenda to include qualitative studies that focus on health and illness. Examples of such studies are Locock and Alexander's (2006) qualitative analysis of male partners' experiences of foetal screening and diagnosis; Oliffe's (2005) analysis of the self-perceived effects on masculinity on men following prostatectomy; Smith and Sparkes' (2005) study of men with spinal injuries; and Gough and Conner's (2006) appraisal of barriers to healthy eating among a sample of men. There has also been a research interest in men's experiences of help-seeking behaviour (O'Brien *et al.* 2005). O'Brien *et al.* (2005) found that while men did tend to position themselves within a discourse of reluctance to avail themselves of help, there were cases which contradicted this trend; however, the researchers note that when help-seeking was invoked, it tended to be for the purposes of facilitating the performance of traditional masculine roles.

Applications to understandings of healthcare

We will consider how feminist theory is brought to bear in understanding healthcare in relation to three interrelated issues:

- The gendered social organization of healthcare.
- Gender issues in healthcare interactions.
- The women's health movement.

The gendered social organization of healthcare

Prior to the 1970s, the gendered patterning in the organization of healthcare was not problematized in academic writings in the manner in which it has been since the advent of feminist analyses. Most accounts of gendering in the social organization of the health services have focused on the relationship between nursing and medicine.

One of the earliest gender analyses of the social organization of health work was Eva Gamarnikow's (1978) account of the sexual division of labour in the work of nurses and doctors. Gamarnikow equated the power dynamics of the nurse–doctor–patient relationship with that of the patriarchal family with the physician wielding the most power. Gamarnikow's work tends towards socialist feminism as she connects the gender division of labour between nurses and physicians to the capitalist mode of production. Gamarnikow argued that the gender division of labour separated all aspects of work into male or female components, and subordinated 'female' tasks to 'male tasks'. She notes that:

> In paid employment within capitalism [woman's] relationship to social production is on one level determined by the limits posed by the sexual division of labour. Any analysis seeking an explanation for the fact that women's work under capitalism is different from men's – both within marriage or the domestic mode of production and in wage labour in the capitalist mode of production – must unquestionably address itself to the pervasiveness of patriarchal relations. (Gamarnikow 1978: 189–190)

While it was obvious that the majority of nurses were female and the majority of physicians male, this gendered arrangement tended to be explained through the notion of complementary roles. Wicks succinctly sums up the shift in interpretation in the relationship when it began to be perceived with a feminist lens:

> When feminist theory arrived on the scene in the 1970s, it shone like a beacon onto the nurse/doctor relationship and illuminated the unequal and often exploitative power relations which underpinned the ostensibly complementary gender dimension of the division of labour. It raised vital questions such as who gives the orders and who takes them, who does the stimulating work and who does the drudge work, and who gets paid more and who gets paid less. (Wicks 1998: 4)

The construction of caring as 'drudge' work as suggested in Wicks' quotation above was characteristic of 70s feminism where the focus was on gaining economic independence and breaking down traditional gender roles. Following developments (and indeed theoretical fissures) in feminist thinking, many contemporary feminist approaches attempt to highlight the value of caring work and the need to reward it adequately (Oakley 1993), an issue to which we will return a little further on.

Much feminist work and indeed mainstream sociology of health and illness has focused on the notion of 'medical dominance' whereupon medicine is deemed to largely determine the work of others in the organization of healthcare because of the medical control over diagnosis and prescribing (see Chapter 2). The decision-making capacity of nurses has been theorized as predominantly informal insofar as the decisions they make can be overruled should medical authority re-assert itself (Walby and Greenwell 1994, Porter 1995a, Wicks 1998). Davies (1995) teases out this notion of medical dominance in relation to the organizational culture of masculinity. She notes the manner in which gender shapes roles and relationships in organizations, including those delivering healthcare:

> Whatever the organization or sector of activity under consideration, it is more than likely that positions in the highest echelons will be almost exclusively occupied by men and that 'support' functions will be the preserve of women. It will be men who carry out the work labelled 'managerial' and women who do the work labelled 'clerical' [...]. No matter what the sector, the higher you go, the fewer the women, so that the hierarchy of pay, status and reward matches the hierarchy between the sexes...a five-year-old can with confidence and ease reel off lists of women's jobs. It will not be a perfect representation of what the latest census figures will reveal, but it is likely to be a strikingly close approximation. (Davies 1995: 45)

Davies' argument is that gender is at the very core of organizational culture, where a masculine logic underpins the workings of the organization. This culture sustains as superior the detached, impersonal and objective characteristic of medicine, while simultaneously relegates as secondary the caring work of nurses. James' (1989) earlier analysis also highlighted gendering in the organizational culture, arguing that the workplace was concerned with economic production and associated with men, while personal feelings linked to women were expected to be confined to the realm of the home. Porter's (1992) analysis of relations between nurses and doctors in a hospital in Northern Ireland indicated that while gender continued to be an issue in the relationship between the two parties, its effects were being moderated by an increasing proportion of women in medicine. Female nurses in his study were aware of the impact their gender had on such relations.

A further area where feminist theory mediates the organization of healthcare relates to the feminist ethic of care, referred to in the earlier section on principles of feminist theory. This ethic of care has been applied in clinical contexts such as in the management of chronic pain (Ferrell 2005), and is also advocated in public health delivery (Roberts and Reich 2002). Furthermore, feminist theorists have contributed to the problematization of bioethics by highlighting its narrow, individualistic construction of personhood and autonomy in favour of a relational approach to autonomy in which individual decision-making is located within a nexus of social relations and situations (MacKenzie and Stoljar 2000). The feminist ethic of care also mediates feminist analyses of the social organization of caring in attempting to uncover and make visible the work involved in *informal* caring for older and disabled relatives, hitherto not even considered to be work (Burton 1975, Glendinning 1983, Ungerson 1987, Lewis and Meredith 1988). Such analyses indicate that informal caring is not predominantly undertaken by families, but rather by women in families. A more recent account of women's caring role for a child with special feeding needs has invoked a feminist poststructuralist position in exploring the manner in which mothers engage in surveillance practices of their mothering against a background of normative constructions of motherhood (Craig and Scambler 2006). Already we can see overlaps between the issue of how healthcare is gendered in its organization, and how gender pervades the type of care that is delivered, the subject of the next section.

Gender issues in healthcare interactions

Since the 1970s, feminist writers have attempted to make visible the manner in which gender permeates the delivery of healthcare. Thus, it is not merely the structuring of relations between health workers that is of interest to feminist writers (the focus of the preceding sub-section) – there is also a concern with understanding issues of gender when women interface with the health services. In unpacking interactions between women and healthcare providers, it is often difficult to disentangle the nature of the encounters from how health and illness are socially constructed by health workers and in society more generally. To clarify, in an earlier section, we referred to Chesler's (1972) study of how normative constructions of femininity influence the interpretation of behaviours (e.g., passivity viewed as normal for women). In turn, the medical construction of illness or normative categories of behaviour can spill over to mediate healthcare interactions. Feminist critics of biomedicine tend to view the medical profession as an elite, patriarchal institution in whose everyday practices gender inequalities are played out. Feminist researchers have hitherto drawn attention to the construction of women in healthcare encounters as passive, submissive, unintelligent, deviant or hypochondriac (Macintyre 1977, 1991, Oakley 1980, Lillrank 2003, Åsbring and Närvänen 2003, Werner and Malterud 2003, Werner et al. 2004). The notion of the 'clinical gaze' (Foucault, 1973; see Chapter 4) has been taken up by feminist sociologists and health activists to critique the medical appropriation of women's bodies (Davis 2007).

A key area of healthcare where much feminist critique centres is that of male-dominated obstetrics, and in particular, on the power that obstetricians wield in framing all normal pregnancies and births as risky (Murphy-Lawless 1998). The feminist critique is that this results in all pregnancies and births being medicalized, an excessive use of technology, and women being reduced to reproductive machines dependent upon technical assistance to give birth (Oakley 1980). Critics of the medicalization of childbirth provide evidence that the bulk of the interventions do not make births safer (Coalition for Improving Maternity Services 2007); rather medical scientific developments have a spurious relationship with the historical reduction in perinatal mortality. They propose instead that improved mortality rates have been brought about through an improvement in living standards (Tew 1998).

The use of New Reproductive Technologies (NRTs) – 'IVF, embryo transfer, sex presentation, genetic engineering of embryos, cloning and more' (Spallone 1989: 14) – has also been debated among feminists. Some feminists – those who believe that women's reproductive capacity impedes women's freedom and independence – interpret NRTs in a positive way on the basis that this technology liberates women from biological motherhood. Other feminist scholars are sceptical about the real benefits of these technologies for women, proposing instead that they do more for the egos and careers of medical scientists than for the women on whom they are applied, given the low success rates in terms of resulting in the live birth of a baby. They also problematize the notion of women's bodies being controlled by male medical technocrats (for a useful account of these debates, see Kent 2000). Central to this issue is a critique of science and the manner in which science is presented as sets of 'facts' rather than as socially produced knowledge constituted through discursive practices and sets of social relationships (see Webster 1991 and Chapter 7).

While gender-focused studies of healthcare have tended historically to concentrate on relations between physicians and female patients, recent studies have also focused on nurses' and midwives' interactions with their client groups. We can see the influence of feminist theory in how data from some of these studies are analysed (Blackford and Street 2002, McCourt 2006). Blackford and Street's (2002) study offers a good example of the overt utilization of feminist theory to inform the research. The research invoked a feminist praxis approach (an approach that links theory to action) to the study of paediatric nurses supporting women of a non-English-speaking background whose child was hospitalized in an Australian hospital. The researchers are explicit that, in a departure from earlier feminist research, their approach to data analysis did not prioritize gender over ethnicity. The study found that equality-aware nurses supporting the mothers of the hospitalized children encountered tensions between their own (the nurses) Western feminist values rooted in philosophies of equality in heterosexual relationships and shared parenting, and some women's own acceptance of patriarchal relationships as part of their culture. The notion of reflectivity was part of the process for the nurses, who, in spite of their philosophies of shared parenting, were challenged by their own deep-seated value systems that caused them to question situations where care was not provided by the mother. Blackford and Street (2002) argue that nurses were following a liberal feminist agenda of sameness, and did not factor cultural differences into their care. Attempts at facilitating women to be assertive in the face of patriarchal dominance later came to be viewed by the nurses as a type of cultural imposition at a time of heightened stress for these women.

McCourt (2006) provides an account of how the midwifery ideals of equality, autonomy and woman-centred care are not always in evidence in midwifery practice. The study, a micro-analysis of communication between midwives and women, found that interactions within a health institution were more hierarchical and less woman-centred than those that occurred between the two parties in the community. Of the institutionally based interactions between midwives and the women, McCourt concluded,

In many ways, the data were strikingly reminiscent of earlier work on professional–client interaction, even that focused on doctors and their patients. The analysis suggests that greater attention to the issues of power and hierarchy, with consequent structural changes, are needed in order to achieve genuine health service reform. (McCourt 2006: 1317)

McCourt indicates that the structural organization of the institution impacts upon the type of communication between midwives and women. Her conclusion rests easily with Davies' (1995) notion, referred to above, that the bureaucratic masculine logic underlies organizational culture and permeates the work of those working within it.

The women's health movement

An important manifestation of the application of feminist theory to understandings of healthcare is the impact upon healthcare of the women's health movement. The women's health movement constitutes a field of feminist activism that has attempted to make policy and practical changes regarding many of the issues debated by feminist theorists. In the early 1970s, reproductive rights dominated the agenda with concerns about abortion rights, birth control and maternity care. The publication of radical texts such as *Our Bodies Ourselves* (Phillips and Rausen 1971) was an example of how theoretical debates about women's bodies and resistance to medical definitions of female embodiment were filtered down to the general population. Women were encouraged to develop a knowledge of their own bodies as a means to resist narrow medical constructions of the female body and to facilitate women to have greater control over their own bodies. In the more recent period, the range of issues with which the women's health movement is concerned has expanded to encompass a variety of health concerns associated with poverty, racism and the environment for women around the globe (Davis 2007).

Although the women's health movement is linked with feminism, some feminist theorists are critical of the movement's heavy focus on women's bodies and reproductive functions, and draw parallels between it and the biomedical gaze (Birke 1999, Haraway 1999, Kuhlmann and Babitsch 2002).

Conclusion and new directions for healthcare

In this chapter, we have highlighted the fissured characterization of feminist theory in view of its multiple internal theoretical perspectives. Like much social theorizing, feminist theory is mediated by a variety of other modes of conceptualization that can result in quite diverse positions. As indicated in this chapter, applying feminist theory to health research is not a straightforward business; however, it offers those engaged in healthcare a different lens with which to view the world. Those wishing to dismiss feminist theory in an era of post-feminist discourses that suppose that women have achieved what they were looking for are challenged to engage with contemporary contributions to this genre of work and to offer well-argued counter-claims before consigning it to the theory archives.

In conclusion, one might ask what feminist theory offers in terms of understanding health and healthcare over and above other theoretical possibilities, and where does it go from here? Healthcare researchers that adopt an explicit feminist stance often draw attention to how knowledge developed from a feminist perspective has the potential to bring about fundamental changes in understanding healthcare and its delivery (see Inhorn and Whittle 2001, Turris 2005). They particularly identify the way in which feminist research strives to address the diverse and interrelated forms of oppression based on gender, ethnicity and class, although the relationship between these social divides is variously interpreted across the broad church of feminisms. For example, Inhorn and Whittle (2001: 558) argue that a feminist framework could 'decenter' epidemiology 'from its masculinist, white, Euro-American axis of privilege to allow for more democratic, egalitarian and participatory ways of knowing and using knowledge'. Turris (2005: 295) similarly proposes a reconceptualization of the traditional measurement of 'patient satisfaction', which she argues, can be represented more fully if explored using a feminist lens. The benefits, she proposes, are that a feminist framework sensitizes the researcher to the voices of those normally excluded, situates the knowledge in the context where it is generated, makes visible gender power relations in healthcare and has the potential to create more humanistic models for healthcare delivery. Porter (1995b: 1133) refers to the potential of feminist theory to inform nursing work, whereupon it offers nurses a set of values that afford women 'their full humanity' and fosters an appreciation of personal experience as a knowledge form. Standpoint feminists argue that the knowledge they produce is more valid than that of conventional research (a position challenged by postmodern feminists as indicated earlier) because they begin from the perspectives of women, and thus open up knowledge forms hitherto concealed behind conventional and predominantly quantitative research methodologies.

With regard to new directions for research, recent work in feminist theory has begun to re-evaluate the place of biology in the enduring debate about how to interpret the female body (Davis 2007). Writers such as Lynda Birke (2003), while cautioning against falling back into dualistic, essentialist thinking, have called for a reconsideration of the place of biology in theorizing the body. As far as bringing back the biological to feminist theory is concerned, Birke (2003) suggests that it is critical that biology is brought back to social sciences and to feminism in a particular way that acknowledges biology as a component of social engagement and not as an *a priori* presocial entity upon which the social dimension is built. According to Birke's proposed perspective, there is a shift from seeing biology as a given foundation upon which the social interacts to a focus on how social interactions influence the biological process of the body *and viceversa*.

This rescuing of biology is likely to be welcomed by feminist health researchers, since the notion of a disembodied body (Davis 2007) represented in feminist postmodern work is problematic for studying experiences of pain, impairment and suffering (see Williams and Bendelow 1998). Future research is also likely to continue focusing on embodied experiences from women's standpoint, in spite of the postmodern perception of women's experiences as the product of cultural discourses and institutional practices as indicated earlier in this chapter. The way forward, as proposed by a number of feminist thinkers (Kruks 2001, Davis 2007), is to begin from the experiences of women, but to theorize these in relation to cultural discourses and institutional arrangements and the socio-political contexts in which they arise.

CHAPTER 7

Science and Technology Studies, Health and Healthcare

Introduction

Since the late nineteenth century, medicine has been firmly wedded to the natural sciences and technological development has played a key role in the institutional organization and values of medicine. Despite this historical relationship, the sociology of science and technology and the sociology of medicine have, to a large extent, remained distinct areas of theory and research. This chapter introduces the reader to the main tenets of what has become known as Science and Technology Studies (STS) by tracing its theoretical lineage to the sociology of science and the turn towards *social contructivism* in the sociology of scientific knowledge (SSK). The social constructivist theories that we introduce in this chapter differ from the theory of *social constructionism* found in the classical work of Berger and Luckmann (1966). In that work (as discussed in Chapter 3), Berger and Luckmann attempt to bring phenomenological and social structural views together in understanding how *social actions* are both shaped by and shape society. *Constructionism* is also a term that is widely used in relation to diverse theoretical perspectives that emanate from the sociology of knowledge and stand in critical opposition to positivist notions of science, including feminism (Chapter 6) and poststructuralism (Chapter 4). In this chapter the precepts of STS are identified with reference to a number of distinct theoretical approaches. We begin with the so-called 'Strong Programme' in SSK and its association with what has become known as 'controversy studies', and then move on to discuss the two main *constructivist* theories in STS – namely, the Social Construction of Technology (SCOT) and Actor Network Theory (ANT).

What we mean by 'constructivist' approaches to scientific knowledge and technology will become clearer to the reader in the following section. Finally, we will address a more recent analytical approach that explores the role of expectations in the development of new technologies.

Our beliefs about medical technologies, whether routine or novel, are coloured by our cultural understandings of medicine as a therapeutic enterprise. Following intense public debates and heightened expectations about the role of molecular biology in revolutionizing medicine, as well as changing our understandings of health, there has been a proliferation of social scientific research exploring the social meaning and implications of genetic technologies in healthcare and society more generally. These studies tend to focus on the social consequences of technology and, therefore, fall within what is generally termed the 'social shaping perspective' (Lohan 2000, Sætnan 2000). In the first section of this chapter, we draw out the key distinctions between this approach to technology, which is linked to *structuralist* views of society, and the *contructivist* approaches associated, in particular, with SCOT and ANT. We then go on to explore how STS is applied to the study of molecular science and genetic technologies in medicine and how this can contribute to our understanding of how the future of health and healthcare is being mobilized by the expectation that medical genetics heralds a paradigm shift.

Principles of science and technology studies

The authority of science lies in the modern belief in 'progress', which equates science with the cumulative technical capacity to harness the natural world for the betterment of humanity. In this sense, science is understood as the foundation of social progress, while technology is commonly understood as the application of scientific knowledge. In the classical philosophy of science, the social and the scientific are conceived of as two separate spheres of activity. Moreover, knowledge of the natural sciences is not amenable to sociological investigation because, as the classical view holds, scientific knowledge is determined by the natural world (Knorr-Cetina and Mulkay 1983). The classical philosophy of science underscores what has become a core belief system within the scientific community and popular representations of science, that is, the idea that science is a privileged type of knowledge, which operates in its own autonomous sphere uninfluenced by social factors. This view holds that science, unencumbered by the social world in the form of social values or subjective preferences and biases, is able to engage in objective and systematic observations of the natural world. Stemming from this classical legacy is the longstanding, *positivist* view of the nature of scientific theories as unmediated empirical observations of the natural world, which places much store in the objectivity of the scientific method for the production of knowledge. While the sociology of knowledge from its inception sought to explain the social processes by which knowledge is produced – how knowledge reflects the social interests, dominant culture and political beliefs of those who produce it – it continued to hold to the idea that the natural sciences were different to other systems of knowledge and belief. This classical view was carried on in the sociology of science under the influence of Robert Merton (1910–2003).

Science as a social institution

In the same functionalist tradition as Parsons (Chapter 1), Merton (1968, 1973) sought to explain how the function of science in contributing to the progress of society is socially structured by institutional norms. Merton's focus was on understanding science as a social institution. While he did not question the validity of scientific knowledge, he did accept that the problems that science addresses are influenced by the wider socio-political and economic context (Aronowitz 1988). However, as Knorr-Cetina and Mulkay (1983: 11) observe, the social context of science was seen as something that could be investigated as additional to, but separate from, the 'technical core of science'. Merton insisted that the democratic values underpinning the norms of the institution of science ensure that the content of scientific knowledge is safeguarded against social interests. His theory outlined four norms, which he took as intrinsic to the social structure and regulation of modern science. He referred to these as 'universalism', 'communism', 'disinterestedness' and 'organized scepticism'. First, science is orientated towards universalism whereby scientific claims are judged on the basis of 'preestablished impersonal criteria' rather than the 'personal or social attributes' of the claim makers (Merton 1968: 607). Second, 'communism' refers to the ethos of the scientific community, which promotes the common ownership of knowledge. Third, the integrity of science depends on scientists taking a disinterested position with respect to both their method of evaluation and findings (by disinterested, he means having no axe to grind, rather than not being interested); and, finally, the scientific community subjects new findings to critical appraisal. If the scientific method represents the cognitive framework for ensuring standards for the production of scientific knowledge, Merton's norms of scientific behaviour presents a view of science as a well-regulated enterprise (Sismondo 2004). Critics, however, point out that these norms are the very terms in which scientists represent themselves in claiming authority over other systems of knowledge, and that they have greater explanatory power as ideological resources for scientists in pursuing their own interests (Sismondo 2004). Though how well being described as communities would have gone down with mid-twentieth-century American scientists is a matter of conjecture!

The sociology of science began to undergo a more critical moment in the late 1960s and 1970s, as the double-edged nature or Janus face of science and technology as the source of both human emancipation and domination began to figure in political and intellectual debates. Part of the context in which this more critical attitude began to take shape was the growth of Big Science (nuclear power, military technology and biotechnology) and the emergence of oppositional social movements. A counter-movement within the scientific community also developed, influenced by the new social movements, to highlight the way that science was being politically misused in the interests of power. However, this position continued to hold to the ideal of the scientific method and, hence, a positivist understanding of science (David 2005). From the perspective of Marxist and some feminist accounts, power relations reflecting class- and gender-based interests structure science as a social institution. From within this critique, science may be deemed ideologically self-serving when it seeks to rationalize dominant power structures or its own vested interests by placing itself beyond critique. The social shaping perspective – emanating from those critiques of how science as an institution is influenced by external interests – began to focus on the social, political and ideological values that drive science and technology in order to understand the social consequences arising for society. In this somewhat simplified characterization of the development of a more critical approach towards the institution of science, it must be mentioned that both Marxist and feminist social theory have been the main opponents of positivism within the social sciences, arguing that the only valid form of knowledge is that which seeks to transform oppressive structures in society.

The sociology of scientific knowledge

The sociology of scientific knowledge (SSK) was a critical point for the emergence of STS. It marked a shift in focus from understanding science as a social institution to a concern with the content of scientific knowledge and beliefs. Many accounts of SSK begin with Thomas Kuhn's *The Structure of Scientific Revolutions* (1962), and the translation and republication of Ludwig Fleck's ([1935] 1979) study on the modern concept of syphilis. Fleck argued that scientific knowledge is more or less a closed system, so that scientific observations are made, conceptualized and explained within a framework that is consistent with the dominant knowledge system within a scientific community (Aronowitz 1988). Kuhn defined these closed systems as 'paradigms'. A paradigm provides a cognitive framework or worldview in which problems are selected, and those educated and socialized within a scientific community follow a standard repertoire of methodologies and theories and, therefore, particular ways of seeing and interpreting the natural world. Scientific communities undergo a crisis when anomalies and problems can no longer be solved within the theoretical terms of the dominant paradigm. Innovative ideas account for the problems or anomalies in the old paradigm (note, not the problems revealed by the natural world) and create a new vision or paradigm shift or, in Kuhnian terms, a revolution. While sociologists disagree as to whether Kuhn's theory was a radical or conservative thesis on science, Sismondo (2004) insists that it challenged what had been the standard view of scientific knowledge as accumulative, progressive and universal in its orientation, and it became the turning point for the sociology of science.

Having discussed the shift in focus from science as a social institution to science as a cognitive system, it is time now to look at how constructivism emerged as a methodological tool for understanding science as a socially produced system of knowledge. We contrast two different constructivist approaches to the social production of scientific knowledge and go on to link these to the two dominant approaches to the social construction of technology. Because these ideas are quite complex and we can only give cursory attention to some of the core ideas that have shaped STS, at the end of this section we include a diagram (Figure 7.1) sketching the terrain of the ideas that we cover in this section.

**FIGURE 7.1 Overview of Sociology of Science
                and Technology**

Sociology of Science   Sociology of Knowledge Merton (1968, 1973)   Mannheim (1936) The Structure of Scientific Revolutions (T. Kuhn 1962) Sociology of Scientific Knowledge (SSK) 'The Strong Programme'   Laboratory Studies D. Bloor ([1976] 1991)   Latour and Woolgar ([1979] 1986) Science & Technology Studies Social Construction of Technology (SCOT)   Actor Network Theory Bijker *et al.* ([1987] 1990)   (ANT) Callon ([1987] 1990) Latour (1987) Law ([1987] 1990) Sociology of Technological Expectations van Lente (1993) Brown *et al.* (2000) Hedgecoe and Martin (2003)

Constructivist approaches to scientific knowledge

The first approach that we look at was developed by the Edinburgh School of Scientific Knowledge, which has become known as the 'Strong Programme'. The reason for this is that it seeks to explain scientific beliefs as an outcome of social relations following, in particular, the work of David Bloor (Sismondo 2004, David 2005). Bloor ([1976] 1991) sees all knowledge as socially mediated and insists that scientific knowledge has no privileged status in this respect. As Pinch and Bijker ([1987] 1990) explain, the epistemological privilege afforded to science is a matter of culture rather than something special to scientific knowledge itself. In this sense, SSK eschews epistemological certainty for epistemological relativism. Bloor insists that sociology should seek explanations for the origins of and consensus about the validity of knowledge claims rather than taking a stance on the truth or falsity of such claims. In other words, sociologists should apply the same explanatory weight to alternative beliefs within science. The Strong Programme shows how scientific knowledge is constructed by focusing on how, within the scientific community, consensus is achieved about which knowledge claims will be accepted as universal truths. This perspective is associated with the 'interest model', which directs its empirical focus to knowledge disputes within science (hence, this approach is also known as 'controversy studies'). As Bijker *et al.* point out:

> Controversies offer a methodological advantage in the comparative ease with which they reveal the interpretative flexibility of scientific results. Interviews conducted with scientists engaged in a controversy usually reveal strong and differing opinions over scientific findings. ([1987] 1990:27)

But what are the mechanisms by which a particular knowledge claim becomes accepted over others? In contrast to the social shaping perspective (mentioned above) that emphasizes the influence of external social interests (such as capitalist and patriarchal interests) in shaping scientific knowledge, controversy studies look inside the institution of science to determine how the internal interests of scientists themselves and the resources that they can mobilize determine what truth claims become part of the scientific consensus where evidence is in dispute (David 2005). As Barnes (1999) points out, empirical studies of both public and internal science controversies show that experts put their own specific construction on reality depending on their different traditions. Where one body of knowledge becomes more favoured than another in such controversies, Barnes argues,

> ...such a preference is likely to reflect not any alleged degree of correspondence with reality of the favoured expertise but rather contingent, sociologically interesting factors like the perceived authority of one tradition of expertise as opposed to another, or the perceived extent of consensus amongst the expert carriers of the tradition, or the perceived disinterest of the experts in question [...]. (1999: 55)

A key critique of this approach is that it does not connect the play of internal interests within the scientific enterprise to wider social interests operating in the cultural, social and economic context within which science and technology also operate. In defence of this constructivist approach, we may argue that the opening up of scientific knowledge to systematic sociological observation requires a more micro-level approach to the internal mechanisms within science.

However, this perspective does not preclude a macro-level approach linking internal interests to prevailing social structures.

The second approach to understanding science as a socially produced system of knowledge is contained in Latour and Woolgar's ([1979] 1986) ethnographic studies of scientific practices, otherwise known as 'laboratory studies' (Knorr-Cetina 1983, Latour 1983). This work represents a contrasting perspective to the Strong Programme and controversy studies. Rather than seeking to develop explanatory theories about the social processes underlying scientific knowledge claims, this approach focuses on producing thick descriptions of routine technical scientific practices (including scientific writing) (Knorr-Cetina and Mulkay 1983). In Latour's words (1983: 159, original emphasis) the focus is on '...*the very content* of what is being done inside laboratories'. Like the Strong Programme, this approach argues that scientific knowledge is not the unmediated representation of the reality of the natural world. From this perspective, scientific knowledge is socially constructed to the extent that it is contingent on how scientists manipulate nature in terms of both the tools that they use and how they transform the material forces that they work on into scientific objects and resources. The construction of scientific knowledge, from this perspective, refers to what scientists do in manipulating nature and having their ideas taken up. Knorr-Cetina (1983: 117) insists that both of these constructivist approaches are more 'complementary' than 'contradictory'. The implications of this theory, however, depend on different readings: for example, does it imply that scientific facts and objects are wholly socially constituted or constructed (in the postmodernist sense of fictional accounts that deny the existence of underlying structures)? Does it imply that science discovers the properties of the natural world and is, therefore, closer to a naïve realist position? Or does it imply that science explores the properties of the natural world in a manner that is mediated by social processes, which is closer to a critical realist position? (See Chapter 5, which elaborates on the distinction between constructivist and realist accounts of the natural and social worlds.)

Constructivist approaches to technology

In the area of technology studies, the version of social constructivism associated with the Strong Programme has been influential on an approach known as the 'social construction of technology' (SCOT) (Bijker *et al.* ([1987] 1990). With the same epistemological relativist perspective of the Strong Programme, SCOT insists that technology is neither linear in its development nor driven by its own inherent technologic (the logic dictated by technical properties), but is socially shaped. At this point, we need to distinguish again between those approaches that are constructivist and those perspectives that are more structuralist in their understanding of how technology is socially shaped. The reader is reminded that in our opening comments and in the discussion above on science as a social institution, we referred to the latter approach as the 'social shaping perspective'. Both these approaches are defined in opposition to what is commonly referred to as the 'determinist' view of technology or technological determinism. The technological determinist standpoint is premised on two key assumptions. First, technologies are fixed at the point of invention by their technical properties and, therefore, are autonomous from society. Second, the internal logic of how the technology works will determine its uses and effects and, therefore, its impact on society. Both the social shaping and constructivist perspectives challenge these assumptions. Describing the social shaping approach and its immanent critique to technological determinism, Sætnan writes,

> The interpretation of Nature's capacities, the selection of which capacities to exploit technologically, the design of technological artefacts to do so – all are outcomes of social processes and social choices. Technological artefacts are made precisely for social (and thereby also political) reasons, in order to achieve certain social effects.... given the current social structure, who has the power to shape technology and thereby reshape (or, more likely, maintain the current shape of) society? (2000: 3–4)

However, the social shaping perspective has been criticized for replacing technological determinism with structural determinism (Lohan 2000, Sætnan 2000) – the idea that the impact of technology follows the intentional designs of vested interests, and the interests that come into play are predetermined by the underlying structures of power in society.

In contrast, SCOT places much greater emphasis on the technical and social contingencies that are at play in the design, development and uptake of technology, and conceives of technology as a heterogeneous network of technical and social elements or 'socio-technical ensembles' (Bijker 1995). Just as controversy studies are concerned with the 'interpretative flexibility' of scientific facts, SCOT asks why a particular technological option becomes stabilized as the technology of choice over competing technological options. In order to answer this question, SCOT focuses on the way that different social groups (including innovators and prospective users) negotiate their different definitions of the problems to be solved by technology, whether or not these are of a strictly social or technical kind and, in turn, how this determines the technical options that are pursued and the physical design and use of the technology. Different social groups (reflecting their different socio-cultural and political situations) will have different interests and capacities to mobilize resources in favour of particular definitions of a problem and the preferred technological solution. On this point, Sætnan draws out a key distinction between contructivist and structuralist, social shaping perspectives:

> ...constructivist theories of technology [...] hold as a methodologi-
> cal precept that the constitution of social groups relevant to a given
> technological innovation cannot be foreseen. It cannot be known in
> advance what social categories, or what attributes of those categories,
> will be invoked or affected by the process of building a new
> sociotechnology. (Sætnan 2000: 7–8)

The second of the constructivist theories of technology is known as Actor-Network Theory (ANT), and is associated with the work of Latour (1987), Callon ([1987] 1990) and Law ([1987] 1990). ANT is distinguishable from SCOT (and especially from its predecessor) in two main respects. One, it is that it is based on a more radical poststructuralist form of constructivism. Its central point is that one cannot assume at the outset of analysis that certain structural factors are likely to be relevant, such as the scientific or commercial motivation behind the technology – however commonsensical or apparent they may seem. These factors, will only be included if they become apparent in the research (Law [1987] 1990). The obvious retort by structuralists is that one usually cannot see things unless one looks for them. However, advocates of ANT argue that this deliberately agnostic view towards sociological understandings of structures is to develop less conventional explanations of the relations between the social and the technical dimensions of technology. The second distinguishing feature is the concept of the 'actant'. The socio-technical networks that are built in the process of turning novel ideas into more or less stable technologies or artefacts consists of lots of different kinds of elements including human actors and non-human entities such as tools, organisms and money. The approach of ANT is to trace the associations between these various elements; each element only acquires its meaning through its connections with other elements. Of course, not all the elements will be equally significant in shaping the technology but it is a question of the research to show which element is the most important by virtue of how it is connected to the other elements in the network. The most controversial aspect of ANT is that it does not accord human actors any special status over non-humans or material objects. The theoretical insight here is that agency ('things acting') is only 'an effect' of the network (Sismondo 2004: 72). In other words, each element only acquires its meaning in relation to its connection to other elements in the network. ANT is not just concerned with the social relations between human actors but the relations between ideas and objects, between humans and non-humans or humans and objects – in other words, all those elements that make up a technology and define how it might be used. This approach acknowledges that technologies do have effects on the social and material world – in this sense, technologies are also actors in networks of relationships (e.g., the mobile telephone has changed the way many of us communicate, where we communicate and what we understand as appropriate communication). However, these technological effects are not necessarily determinate. Rather the effects of technology are also influenced by the way that the particular technical and social properties of a technology are socially interpreted and used. This approach attempts to counterbalance two previously dominant understandings of technology in society: one that technology determines society (the so called technological determinist approach); the other that society determines technology (the social shaping approach discussed above).

Just as Knorr-Cetina suggests that there is a strong complementarity between the Strong Programme and laboratory studies in SSK, in terms of methodological precepts we may say the same about ANT and SCOT. From the perspectives of both approaches, technology is constructed through the very process of building socio-technical networks (a network made up of social and technical elements). The formation and eventual configuration of a socio-technical network involves the enrolment of various actors, including the scientists and researchers involved in R&D networks, commercial funders, public funders, regulatory agencies, policy makers and prospective users, and the mobilization of the social, technical and economic resources that these actors bring to the network. The network becomes stable over time when there has been a successful alignment of the heterogeneous interests and activities, non-human actors and artefacts in terms of the technological option that is chosen, its physical design, product and market.

Both SCOT and ANT emphasize that the meaning of a particular technological innovation varies in line with the changing configuration of a socio-technical network. As we noted above, different actors within socio-technical networks will also have different resources for mobilizing or constraining support for particular technological options.

'The sociology of technological expectation'

Since uncertainty surrounds most new technologies in relation to technical capabilities, competing visions and the extent to which support from funders, policy makers and the public can be garnered, sociologists have, more recently, begun to explore the role that expectations play in shaping the trajectory of a nascent technology and its possible impact on society. Drawing on the works of van Lente (1993) and Brown *et al.* (2000), Hedgecoe and Martin (2003: 328) refer to this novel theoretical framework, which is incorporated into STS's network concept as the 'sociology of technological expectation'. The expectations about the future possibilities of an emerging technology are by no means self-evident, but as Rappert and Brown (2000: 50) point out, they must be 'mobilized and constructed'. Rather than dismissing the speculative claims made about genetic technologies as mere hype, Hedgecoe and Martin (2003: 328) argue that these claims or the visions that various actors hold about the future possibilities of technology are 'fundamental to the dynamic processes that create new socio-technical networks' and the shape that a technology will eventually take. In this sense visions are 'strategic resources' used to 'mobilize' investment and legitimacy (Hedgecoe and Martin 2003: 341).

In the following sections we focus on some of the burgeoning research that utilizes the theoretical approaches and analytical concepts central to STS in developing a sociological understanding of the complex and contingent dynamics of genetic technology in the field of medicine.

Applications to understandings of health

Elsewhere we have referred to 'medicalization' (see Chapter 6) to describe the process by which more and more aspects of everyday life fall under the jurisdiction of medicine. The terms 'geneticization' (Lippman 1991, 1998) and 'biomedicalization' (Clarke *et al.* 2003) are sociological concepts that define an intensification of the processes of medicalization in the context of the rapid development of molecular genetics and the implications that this holds for how we come to understand our health. While biomedicalization is a political economy concept that refers to the emerging bio-industrial complex supporting the commercialization of genetic research (see Clarke *et al*. 2003), the concept of geneticization is used to signify a more general cultural shift in our cognitive and normative understanding of human behaviour, health and disease. Lippman describes geneticization as:

> ...the ever growing tendency to distinguish people from one another on the basis of genetics; to define most disorders, behaviours, and physiological variations as wholly or in part genetic in origin. It is both a way of thinking and a way of doing, with genetic technologies applied to diagnose, treat, and categorize conditions previously identified in other ways. (1998: 64)

The theme of geneticization is explored in this section in relation to the following:

- The social shaping of genetic, and;
- The geneticization of breast cancer.

Two specific STS case studies that examine breast cancer genetics albeit from different theoretical perspectives.

The social shaping of genetics

The gene has become a cultural icon of the twenty-first century representing what Fox Keller (2000: 132) refers to as 'new forms of biological thought'. For those who follow a social shaping perspective, the powerful cultural grip of 'gene talk' has profound social implications (see various essays in Nelkin and Lindee 1995, Conrad and Gabe 1999, Kaplan 2000, Pilnick 2002). In support of the geneticization thesis,[1] the following evidence is referred to in the literature:

- The shift in emphasis in genetic research from rare hereditary, monogentic diseases to more commonly acquired illness and behavioural disorders.

---

[1] See Hedgecoe (2002) and Novas and Rose (2000) for differently argued critiques of the geneticization thesis.

- A shift in focus in diagnostic testing from actual risk to the probability of risk for late onset disorders.
- The widening scope for population-based genetic screening, for example the creation of population-based DNA databases and the proposal to link these to personal medical records (see Martin 2001).

These developments give rise to novel and complex ethical questions, not least of which concern the commercialization of human biological material and the potential to broaden the scope of population surveillance. In a risk-conscious society, the cultural imperatives of healthism and individualism (also discussed in Chapter 4) are a vehicle for the expectations created about molecular genetics for the future management of health and elimination of disease (Cunningham-Burley and Boulton 2000, Petersen and Bunton 2002, Pilnick 2002). At the same time, the ambiguity felt by both health professionals and patients, and wider public ambivalence about the social value of predictive testing (see, e.g., Cunningham-Burley and Boulton 2000, Kerr and Cunningham-Burley 2000, Turney and Turner 2000, Cox and Starzomski 2004, Taylor 2004) creates lines of resistance.

The geneticization of breast cancer

Since the identification of two susceptibility genes for breast cancer (BRCA1 and BRCA2) in the mid-1990s there has been an exponential growth in predictive cancer genetics, a field that continues to be marked by considerable uncertainty about the clinical and social value of genetic testing. There are a number of reasons for this uncertainty: breast cancer is understood as a complex, multifactorial disease; predictive genetic testing is not focused on either the individual patient or the disease itself, but rather on the genetic risk expressed by the disease and the probability that this risk is shared within a family. A positive test result only indicates a susceptibility to breast cancer; it cannot predict the actual occurrence of the disease or reveal anything about its development. Conversely, a negative test result is not an indication that the individual will not develop the disease in the future and where family analysis indicates a genetic susceptibility, a negative genetic test result does not rule out a genetic mutation and, therefore, is not conclusive as a diagnostic tool. Given that for the vast majority of patients with a strong family history the genetic mutation remains unknown, and given that DNA testing does not lead to an unambiguous individual diagnosis for the relatively small percentage of cases where a genetic mutation is identified, we can see that this technology is marked by considerable uncertainty. How regulatory processes define and deal with these uncertainties will shape the meaning and use of the technology.

Since genetic testing for breast cancer was 'the first genetic testing technology for a common disease' (Parthasarathy 2005: 33) and the first to be widely commercialized, it is an interesting case to examine in relation to the geneticization thesis. In the discussion below, we introduce the reader to two STS research case studies on predictive cancer genetics. Both papers concern the institutional and regulatory networks involved in the delivery of breast cancer predictive testing. The first case study (Williams-Jones and Graham 2003), which follows an ANT approach, analyses the interests and values that are built into predictive testing technology. Resistance to the commercialization of predictive testing is a dominant theme in this paper. This theme is continued in the second paper by Parthasarathy (2005), which adopts a wider approach than ANT and SCOT by exploring how institutional factors in different political cultures influence different interpretations of how predictive testing technology should be used. Both studies demonstrate how the social processes involved in the development of a technology define who should decide eligibility criteria, who should have access to the technology and under what conditions.

Breast cancer genetics: The case of a failed socio-technical network

One of the key ethical concerns about the development of genetic technologies is the commercialization of publicly funded international collaborative research and the leverage that the patenting of genes gives private interests in determining the shape of and access to a technology. Williams-Jones and Graham's study (2003) traces the ethical issues that led to the failure of the US biotech firm Myriad Genetics to have its test taken up as an 'over the counter' kit in the United States. The methodological precept of their approach is that (2003: 279) '[f]ailed networks are [...] often a fruitful place for study, because it is here that the actor networks reveal themselves and the norms and values built into technologies are made apparent'. They argue that an ANT analysis conceiving of genetic tests as actors within a network helps to broaden the scope of ethical analysis beyond concerns with both the psychosocial impact of genetic testing on individuals and families and the wider social concerns about discrimination and stigmatization likely to arise from a negative genetic test.

Myriad's marketing strategies to both patients and physicians emphasize the primacy of genetics in breast cancer; not surprisingly, little attention is given to the ethical implications of testing while genetic information is marketed as a resource for patients to make informed choices about treatment and life planning (Williams-Jones and Graham 2003). As Parthasarathy (2005: 19) notes, 'Myriad treated BRCA testing as a state-of-the-art product that should be available on demand to all women'. The strong consumer orientation of Myriad's marketing strategies is facilitated by US laws, which allow both direct marketing to consumers and access to testing on the direct referral of a physician. In contrast, most European countries provide testing services through public genetic clinics where risk is initially assessed based on family history (Bourret 2005, Parthasarathy 2005). The key resistance to Myriad's over-the-counter test relates to concerns about the difficulty for consumers in interpreting genetic information when clinicians themselves with specialized knowledge face a multitude of difficulties in translating test results into diagnostic certainty. There is also a strong professional consensus that patients should have access to genetic counselling to address the complex issues involved for individuals and their families in relation to the benefits and risks of undertaking a test. Similar concerns arise in relation to Myriad's minimum criterion that access to testing only requires a referral from a physician who may neither have the specialized knowledge nor multi-disciplinary clinical support necessary to interpret genetic data and support patients in the decision to undergo testing. Among patient advocacy groups, there are also concerns about the implications of being labelled 'at risk' and resistance to the commercialization of genetic testing in the context of the uncertainty of the risk conferred by a test (Parthasarathy 2005). There is also strong resistance in countries that provide public genetic clinics and laboratories to Myriad's strategy of commercial monopoly on the basis that it undermines the provision of affordable and equitable public healthcare. Williams-Jones and Graham (2003) conceive of these as competing actor networks because they inscribe different normative values into genetic technology testing. As we shall see, comparative analyses of the institutional features of regulatory processes reveal how competing values are built into technologies.

Breast cancer genetics: Consumer vs. public health values

In comparing the development of genetic testing in the United States and the United Kingdom, Parthasarathy (2005: 32) demonstrates how the 'architecture' of genetic testing is shaped by different institutional factors in different political cultures and how this, in turn, defines the 'roles, rights, responsibilities, and authority' of healthcare providers, health professionals and users. Parthasarathy's (2005) study identifies an important element of Myriad's legal monopolizing strategy, which enabled it to profit immediately from its patients and, at the same time, expand its genomic database on BRCA. In the United States, Myriad mounted a legal challenge to the blurring of the boundaries between research and clinical care in the development of genetic testing in order to shut down testing services provided as part of clinical research protocols. It argued that research protocols that disclosed genetic information to patients were in effect offering a commercial service and were, therefore, violating patenting law. This effectively meant that those participating in clinical research could no longer access genetic information, allowing '...Myriad to control the definition of research and impose its definition of the boundary between research and commercial service' (Parthasarathy 2005: 24). Parthasarathy goes on to observe that as the monopoly provider of BRCA testing, Myriad is able to limit both health professional and consumer choice to its own testing product.

Since Myriad defines itself as a diagnostic laboratory commercially driven by consumer demand, it has distanced itself from the professional ethical and clinical concerns of those who manage illness (Parthasarathy 2005). Public healthcare systems, on the other hand, define genetic testing in the context of providing clinical care, and the provision of services rather than being consumer led, is aimed at identifying all those at risk with a view to prevention and targeting genetic testing at the small percentage of the population defined as high-risk. In this sense, we could argue that public healthcare systems, which require rationalization according to need and professional clinical norms, act as a break on full-scale geneticization driven by public demand for genetic testing for common cancers. Myriad's commercial testing and market monopoly over testing services define genetic testing within a consumer model of health. Within this model, health professionals are mere facilitators enabling 'customers' to access a commercial service for which they pay. As Parthasarathy notes,

The shape of Myriad's BRCA testing service and its aggressive litiga-
tion strategy are not at all surprising in the context of the weak regulation of the clinical aspects of genetic testing and robust intellectual
property regime in the USA. (2005: 32)

In contrast, health professionals in the United Kingdom act as traditional gatekeepers for scarce public health resources. In this system,
Parthasarathy argues, the client is not a customer but is defined as a
traditional patient subject to clinical risk assessment and judgement
in relation to medical need. Once medical need is established within
the threshold of risk determined by national standards in clinical protocols, access to testing is a question of the rights of citizens and not
ability to pay as in the US consumer model.

The conclusions drawn by Parthasarathy's and Williams-Jones and
Graham's studies, albeit from different theoretical perspectives, are
similar. They both draw attention to the wider political and institutional structures that shape technology. While Williams-Jones and
Graham frame their study within an ANT approach and the analytical
concepts that they use are taken from this perspective, in order to
draw out the ethical implications of commercial genetic testing they
point to the wider social, economic, political and cultural contexts
that shape a technology and its ethical controversies.

Applications to understandings of healthcare

The cultural repertoire that has developed around the public communication of genetic research has contributed to the popularization of a
biologically reductive notion of how genes function, as well as mobilizing public expectations about the future of genetic technology. As it
stands, the perceived importance of genetic medicine for the future of
healthcare goes beyond the actual availability of working technologies
(Hedgecoe and Martin 2003). How health services will take up genetic
technologies is complicated by the uncertainty of the innovative
process itself, not only in terms of its clinical efficacy but also in relation to the uncertainty about its ethical and social implications
(Rappert and Brown 2000). Notwithstanding these widely felt uncertainties, the general expectation that genetic technologies will revolu-
tionize healthcare is actively promoted in policy agendas. This is given
practical intent in the role that policy plays in endorsing institutional
links between academic research and industry to support technological

transfer and commercial exploitation (see Martin and Kaye 2000). For these reasons, Rappert and Brown (2000) argue that public policy is central to the configuration and stabilization of socio-technical networks that support particular technological options. As we have seen, the previous case studies above also support this view. The following discussion focuses on a number of case studies that explore how expectations are mobilized as strategic resources to garner support for particular technological options. The substantive studies that we discuss in some detail involve:

• The case of genetic diagnostics, and;
• The case of pharmacogenetics.

Mobilizing expectations: The case of genetic diagnostics

In their comparative study of the innovatory dynamic of genetic diagnostics and telemedicine, Rappert and Brown (2000: 66) note that '[f]or the former, revolutionary promise plays a certain role as a resource that can mobilize the preparedness of the market and the momentum of the configuration'. In their analysis, this 'revolutionary repertoire' serves to enrol various actors into collaborative networks to sustain a future vision for genetic diagnostics and, in that process, create niche markets. Their study develops a four-dimensional analytical scheme for understanding how the institutional and structural conditions of a particular network create or limit the opportunity for expectations to influence how an innovation will be taken up. The first dimension relates to the expectations that characterize the agenda of the science and technology. In relation to genetic diagnosis, the 'revolutionary motif' is linked to the newness and embryonic stage of the science and technology of genetics. The shared vision held by key actors is based on the promise of improving health and eliminating disease, which appeals to patients' hopes. However, the opportunity for sustaining this shared vision is limited by the ethical concerns thrown up by genetic medicine and, in turn, the uncertainty that this raises for regulatory politics. In addition, there are significant ambiguities and tensions about the governance of public/private R&D collaborations, which are ostensibly about guiding science towards the public good of health. The key source of tension here is between industry's interest in the patenting and commodification of genetic data and the mandate of public policy to protect patients and patient confidentiality. As we noted in the previous section, this tension generates resistance amongst various types of users, including the state, health professionals and end-users (patients and potential patients).

The next dimension is the configuration of the network. Here, the authors emphasize the role of large pharmaceutical companies who are the most powerful actors driving genetic technology and the market scope for smaller and medium-sized biogenetic companies, which has resulted in extensive and durable R&D networks. The architecture of genetic diagnostics and pharmacogenetics (discussed below) follows a similar pattern in the proliferation of smaller biotechnology firms aligned to multinational pharmaceutical companies who invest huge resources in clinical trials and bringing the product to the market. The political legitimacy of the key sector actors, however, depends on enrolling patient and public support, which is beset by problems that go beyond technical concerns. Given the uncertainty surrounding the regulatory environment for genetic medicine, Rappert and Brown point out that the rules that bind the various actors together are under debate and the focus is on developing bioethical policy and protocols so that the technology can be taken up.

The third dimension of their analytical scheme involves the management of the innovation so that the expectations created about genetic diagnosis can shape the responses of individual organizations. There are a number of key features here including the technical uniformity of product standards, the resources of the big players to sustain the long timeframe in launching a product and the emphasis on redefining and creating new needs for market products. Managing innovation in relation to genetic diagnostics is much more difficult for healthcare systems given the demands that new needs create in terms of managing patients and scarce health resources.

Finally, Rapport and Brown (2003: 69) refer to how networks and the organizations within them engage with what they term 'future-oriented coordination' through their participation in formal and informal forums where actors establish their place at the table in the formulation of national policies to support innovation and its uptake.

This study shows that the novelty and uncertainty pertaining to genetic diagnostics limits the opportunities of key actors to mobilize for an alignment of all actors into a stable sociotechnical network. Ethical issues have an important role to play because of the difficulty of mobilizing support for those technologies, which prove to be too controversial. For this reason, as Cunningham-Burley and Kerr (1999) note, it is increasingly difficult for scientists and clinicians to avoid public and professional recognition that genetic technologies raise wider social implications. Martin (2001) also argues that the incorporation of ordinary citizens into various advisory committees on the ethical and social implications of genetics may be viewed as a policy strategy to enrol public support for genetic science. The pharmaceutical industry is also actively involved in supporting and funding patients' groups and so it plays a powerful role in aligning the supply and demand dynamics within social-technical networks.

Mobilizing expectations: That case of pharmacogenetics

Pharmacogenetics (the study of genetic variation in drug response), or what is more recently termed 'pharmocogenomics' (the development of drugs that can be adapted to an individual's genetic make-up), has become a key part of the future-oriented investment strategies of the big pharmaceutical companies and is flagged as the next big public/private research collaboration. This area of research is now seen as more promising in terms of the treatment of common diseases than earlier expectations held out for gene therapy. As Martin's (1999) ANT study of gene therapy argues, the definition of more and more common diseases such as cancer as genetic and the prospect that this initially held out for gene therapy paved the way for commercial interest in genetic drug-based therapies. While the pharmaceutical industry is poised to mobilize the future of pharmacogenetics and is increasingly involved in the collection of DNA samples as a core activity of clinical trials, a significant gap still exists between the promise of the technology and actual commercial products (Hedgecoe and Martin 2003).

In a study exploring the role of expectations in the development of pharmacogentics, Hedgecoe and Martin (2003) identify two visions that dominate the scientific and clinical literature. The first vision is based on the genetic basis of drug metabolism, which has been established since the late 1950s. The basic scientific premise behind this vision is that variation in an individual's genetic make-up correlates with a drug's efficacy or toxicity. While drugs may be effective for a majority of patients with a specific disease, for a small or substantial minority the same drugs at standard dosages may prove ineffective or dangerously toxic. The anticipated benefits of this vision are that both individual patients and healthcare systems will gain from a reduction in deaths and in the cost of health implications arising from adverse drug reactions (ADR). The expectation created to mobilize the interest and resources of pharmaceutical companies is that pharmacogenetics will allow the industry to re-capture drugs that have failed in the later stages of clinical trials by creating niche markets based on the genetic profile of sub-population patient groups, as well as tailoring drug trials to target population groups that are more likely to respond positively to a drug (also see Snedden 2000). Hedgecoe and Martin argue that since a genetic test for drug reaction does not involve disease diagnosis or prognosis, it does not raise the level of ethical concern identified with the second vision. This vision is much more radical in its proposition that pharmacogenetics will tailor drugs to the underlying disease mechanisms operating at molecular level for individual patients. A genetic test to identify a gene marker for a disease that may indicate a particular drug response could double up as a prognosis for the type and severity of a disease that a patient might develop.

While a common adage to be found in discussions of bioethics is that it is constantly on the back foot trying to catch up with a technology that outpaces public understanding and ethical and legal frameworks, Hedgecoe and Martin (2003) show that bioethics is increasingly integral to the way that scientists construct their vision in mobilizing expectations to capture the future of technology. Part of the context for understanding why researchers and industry seek to deploy a bioethical discourse in the construction of their visions for technology is that bioethics has increasingly become part of the institutional context that shapes policy discourse and regulatory frameworks in the context of biotechnology. Since scientists are clearly aware of the need to enrol public support, those who advocate the ADR vision of pharmacogenetics seek to distinguish it from predictive genetic testing, and hence distance it from the ethical controversies central to public debate on disease diagnostics. Indeed, some commentators argue that pharmacogenetic testing is an ethical imperative to reduce harm to patients. In the case of the second vision where a test for drug reaction may also double as a predictive test for a disease, the gamut of ethical issues raised by genetic testing cannot be ignored. As Møldrup observes (2002: 31), the ethical concerns arising from the expectation that pharmacogenetic drugs will 'become public genetic information markers of an individual's genetic predisposition' is a key point of resistance to the legitimacy of this kind of technology.

In a later published case study of pharmacogenetics, Hedgecoe (2006) further develops the sociology of socio-technical expectation, but within the framework of the SSK and controversy studies. In this study, Hedgecoe focuses on a much-cited, but disputed study (Poirier *et al.* 1995) that claims that there is a pharmacogenetic link between reduced response to the anti-Alzheimer's Disease drug Tacrine for those who carry the *APoE4* allele. The disputed *APoE4*/Tacrine link is at the heart of ethical debates on pharmacogenomics because when a genetic test to predict whether or not that person is a good or bad responder to a drug identifies the presence of the *APoE4* allele, the presence of that gene marker is predicting a risk factor for other family members. Hedgecoe's study shows how a scientific claim can be held within the wider scientific community and promoted as fact in the formulation of health policy even when those researchers and clinicians working within the specialized domain dispute the claim and where there is a strong ethical consensus that predictive genotyping is controversial. Particular actors have specific interests in mobilizing expectations about the future of pharmacogenetics. In the case of those who cite the contested link between *APoE4* and Tacrine as solid evidence of the future of pharmacogenetics in healthcare, particular interests are at play. These include large pharmaceutical companies and biotech firms who have invested heavily in and are core to the pharmacogenomic 'project'. Hedgecoe also notes that pharmacologists and pharmacists also have particular interests in citing the disputed study in creating expectations about the creation of a pharmacogenetically defined healthcare system, since they see an expansion of their role in advising clinicians on prescribing drugs based on patients' genetic profiles.

Conclusion and new directions for healthcare

In summary, social constructivism represents the most radical refutation of naïve realist views in that it rejects the epistemological claim that the nature of an object determines the form of its possible science. Social constructivists, for the most part, insist that constructivism is an epistemological issue not an ontological position – that it is contesting what we can 'know', not what actually exists. This, of course, brings problems in itself. If all forms of knowledge are treated as equally legitimate, then how are the very obvious differences in the status of knowledge claims between experts and lay people or even amongst different specialisms within a given field of expertise to be explained? One answer can be found in Chapter 4, where Foucauldian analysts were seen to argue that this results from the relationship between power and knowledge and the social hierarchies and conflicts found in the production of knowledge. An alternative view can be found in Chapter 5, where we saw a variant of structuralist approaches in the form of critical realism. Thus, we saw in Conrad's critique of the new genetics an argument that the model of genetic determinism was misleadingly partial. Implicit in this argument was the assumption that an appreciation of the complex web of causality, in which genetic information interacts with environmental factors, provides a fuller knowledge of the causes of health and illness than that provided by the new genetics. In other words, it entailed an assumption that there are better and worse ways of knowing about what exists and how it works.

In this chapter, we trace the theoretical linkages between constructivist approaches to scientific knowledge and constructivist approaches to technology. In particular, we link the 'Strong Programme' in SSK to SCOT, and the more radical constructivist position of Latour to ANT. Because the terms 'socially constructed' and 'socially shaped' are often used interchangeably by standpoints that reject the notion of technological determinism, we draw out some basic distinctions between those approaches that are *constructivist* and those perspectives that are more *structuralist* in their understanding of the social process of technological innovation. In the STS case studies discussed in the chapter, these approaches do not preclude one another whether we are looking at the expectations, interests and investments that shape technology, or the form that they eventually take – how they are politically regulated, and embedded in institutional arrangements and practices.

While the various perspectives that make up STS are distinct, they share a number of key ideas in relation to the way that science and technology are socially constructed. These may be summarized as:

- Science and technology are social activities that are, for the most part, interdependent.
- Just as scientific knowledge is open to different and, sometimes, competing interpretations, technologies are not driven by an innate technical logic but are interpretatively flexible.
- Scientific knowledge and technology are socially shaped in the negotiations between diverse actors such as scientists, engineers, clinicians, venture capitalists, policy makers, the public and end users (socio-technical networks).
- Just as the creation of science and technology is not merely technical or solely social in origin, the impact of scientific and technological developments are not determined by their natural or technological properties, nor explained by social structures alone.

STS, for the most part, is an empirically driven enterprise and research tends to be far more eclectic in its interpretation and use of distinct theories. For example, SCOT and ANT are often integrated in case-study methodologies in ways that do not adequately distinguish between the theoretical interpretations of both, and the approach of ANT, in particular, is open to different if not incompatible interpretations. While the perspective of ANT (following Latour) would appear to rule out the idea that sociological analyses can systematically explain the relationship between social power and interests in shaping technology, we saw how Williams-Jones and Graham (2003) argue that social critique is not precluded by empirical studies that adopt this approach. A critique of STS more generally and a charge that can be equally applied to ANT- and SCOT-centred approaches or controversy studies is the failure to address the wider social and political context of science and technology. For example, in our discussion of the applications of STS to understanding health, Parthasarathy (2005) shows how national comparative analyses of genetic technology require much closer attention to the cultural and political contexts that shape technologies. Another general critique of STS that is applied, in particular, to both the Strong Programme and ANT is that it rules out questioning the validity of scientific claims. Williams-Jones and Graham, however, not only show how Myriad's claim that its commercial BRCA test is more accurate than other testing systems is clinically contested, but in highlighting its marketing strategies they develop a strong sociological critique of Myriad's claims. Furthermore, we have shown with reference to the burgeoning research literature on genetic medicine from the perspective of ANT that the effect of socio-technical networks in shaping technology depends on the heterogeneous composition and alignment of the various elements of that network, and the extent to which different social actors can mobilize strategic resources. We are aware of the risk of misrepresenting ANT here,[2] however, even in the substantive case studies discussed in this chapter ANT is interpreted and used in different ways.

Depending on the research focus and scope, different studies will emphasize different elements, social actors and resources. The focus of

---

[2] For a broader resource on how ANT is interpreted and used, see the Actor Network Resource, An Annotated Bibliography, Department of Sociology and Centre for Science Studies, Lancaster University, UK (http://www.comp.lancs.ac.uk/sociology/css/antres.htm, Version 2.13).

References

Acheson, D., Barker, D., Chambers, J., Graham, H., Marmot, M. and Whitehead, M. (1998) *The Report of the Independent Inquiry into Inequalities in Health*. London: The Stationary Office.

Ackerson, B. (2003) Coping with the dual demands of severe mental illness and parenting: The parents' perspective. *Families in Society*, 84(1), 109–118.

Actor Network Resource. An Annotated Bibliography, Department of Sociology and Centre for Science Studies, Lancaster University, UK. http://www/comp. lancs.ac.uk/sociology/css/antres.htm, Version 2.13.

Adam, B., Beck, U. and van Loon, J. (eds) (2000) *The Risk Society and Beyond: Critical Issues for Social Theory*. London: Sage.

Adamson, J. A., Ebrahim, S. and Hunt, K. (2006) The psychosocial versus material hypothesis to explain observed inequality in disability among older adults: Data from the West of Scotland Twenty-07 Study. *Journal of Epidemiology and Community Health*, 60, 974–980.

Adkins, L. (2005) Feminist social theory. In Harrington, A. (eds) *Modern Social Theory: An Introduction*. Oxford: Oxford University Press, 233–251.

Ainsworth-Vaughn, N. (1998) *Claiming Power in Doctor-Patient Talk*. Oxford: Oxford University Press.

Allen, D. (1997) The nursing-medical boundary: A negotiated order? *Sociology of Health and Illness*, 19(4), 498–520.

Almedom, A. M. (2005) Social capital and mental health: An interdisciplinary review of primary evidence. *Social Science and Medicine*, 61(5), 943–964.

Altschuler, A., Somkin, C. P. and Adler, N. E. (2004) Local services and amenities, neighborhood social capital, and health. *Social Science and Medicine*, 59(6), 1219–1229.

American Heart Association. (2007) Facts about women and cardiovascular diseases. http://www.americanheart.org/presenter.jhtml?identifier=2876. January 2, 2007.

Anderson, R. and Bury, M. (eds) (1988) *Living with Chronic Illness: The Experience of Patients and their Families*. London: Unwin Hyman.

Annandale, E. (1998) *The Sociology of Health and Medicine: A Critical Introduction*. Cambridge: Polity Press.

Appel, A. L. and Malcolm, P. (2002) The triumph and continuing struggle of nurse practitioners in New South Wales, Australia. *Clinical Nurse Specialist*, 16(4), 203–210.

Arber, S. and Khlat, M. (2002) Introduction to 'social and economic patterning of women's health in a changing world'. *Social Science and Medicine*, 54(5), 643–647.

Archer, M. (1995) *Realist Social Theory: A Morphogenetic Approach*. Cambridge: University of Cambridge Press.

Archer, M. S. (1988) *Culture and Agency*. Cambridge: Cambridge University Press.

Archer, M. S. (1990) Human agency and social structure: A critique of Giddens. In Clarke, J., Modgil, C. and Modgil, S. (eds) *Anthony Giddens: Consensus and Controversy*. Basingstoke: Falmer Press.

Armstrong, D. (1997) Foucault and the sociology of health and illness: A prismatic reading. In Petersen, A. and Bunton, R. (eds) *Foucault, Health and Medicine*. London and New York: Routledge, 15–30.

Armstrong, D. (2002) Clinical autonomy, individual and collective: The problem of changing doctors' behaviour. *Social Science and Medicine*, 55(10), 1771–1777.

Aronowitz, S. (1988) *Science as Power: Discourse and Ideology in Modern Society*. Basingstoke, Hampshire: Macmillan.

Åsbring, P. and Närvänen, L. (2003) Ideal versus reality: Physicians' perspectives on patients with chronic fatique syndrome (CFS) and fibromyalgia. *Social Science and Medicine*, 57(4), 711–720.

Astell, M. (1694) *A Serious Proposal to the Ladies for the Advancement of Their True and Greatest Interest*. London: Printed for Wilkin [Wing A4063].

Atkinson, P. (1995) *Medical Talk and Medical Work: The Liturgy of the Clinic*. London: Sage.

Atkinson, P. A. (1997) *The Clinical Experience* (2nd edition). Aldershot, UK: Ashgate.

Barker, K. (2004) Self-help literature and the making of an illness identity: The case of fibromyalgia syndrome (FMS). In Conrad, P. (ed.) *The Sociology of Health and Illness: Critical Perspectives* (7th edition). New York: Worth Publishers, 133–150.

Barker, D. J. P. (1998). *Mothers, Babies and Health in Later Life*. Edinburgh: Churchill Livingstone.

Barnes, B. (1999) Biotechnology as expertise. In O'Mahony, P. (ed.) *Nature, Risk and Responsibility: Discourses of Biotechnology*. Basingstoke, Hampshire: Macmillan, 52–66.

Barnett, J. R. and Barnett, P. (2004) Primary healthcare in New Zealand: Problems and policy approaches. *Social Policy Journal of New Zealand*, 21, 49–66.

Barnett, J. R., Barnett, P. and Kearns, R. (1998) Declining professional dominance?: Trends in the proletarianisation of primary care in New Zealand. *Social Science and Medicine*, 46(2), 193–207.

Bartley, M. (2004) *Health Inequality: An Introduction to Theories, Concepts and Methods*. Cambridge: Polity.

Batty, G. D., Morton, S. M., Campbell, D., Clark, H., Davey Smith, G., Hall, M., Macintyre, S. and Leon D. A. (2004) The Aberdeen Children of the

1950s cohort study: Background, methods and follow-up information on a new resource for the study of life course and intergenerational influences on health. *Paediatric and Perinatal Epidemiology*, 18(3), 221–239.

Baum, F. (1999) The role of social capital in health promotion: Australian perspectives. *Health Promotion Journal of Australia*, 9(3), 171–178.

Baum, F., Bush, R., Modra, C., Murray, C., Cox, E., Alexander, K. and Potter, R. (2000) Epidemiology of participation: An Australian Community Study. *Journal of Epidemiology and Community Health*, 54, 414–423.

Beck, C. T. (1992) The lived experience of postpartum depression: A phenomenological study. *Nursing Research*, 41(3), 166–170.

Beck, U. (1992) *Risk Society*. London: Sage.

Becker, H., Geer, B., Hughes, E. C. and Strauss, A. (1961) *Boys in White: Student Culture in Medical School*. New York: New York University Press.

Bejakel, M. and Goldblatt, P. (2006) Introduction. In Bejakel, M., Osborne, V., Yar, M. and Meltzer, H. (eds) *Focus on Health*. An ONS (UK Official National Statistics) publication. Basingstoke: Palgrave Macmillan.

Bell, J., Zimmerman, F. J., Almgren, G. R., Mayer, J. D. and Huebner, C. E. (2006) Birth outcomes among urban African-American women: A multilevel analysis of the role of racial residential segregation. *Social Science and Medicine*, 63(12), 3030–3045.

Bendelow, G. and Williams, S. J. (eds) (1998) *Emotions in Social Life: Critical Themes and Contemporary Issues*. London: Routledge.

Bendelow, G. (1993) Pain perceptions, emotions and gender. *Sociology of Health and Illness*, 15(3), 273–294.

Ben-Shlomo, Y. and Kuh, D. (2002) A life course approach to chronic disease epidemiology: Conceptual models, empirical challenges and interdisciplinary perspectives. *International Journal of Epidemiology*, 31(2), 285–293.

Bensing, J. M., Verhaak, P. F. M., van Dulmen, A. M. and Visser, A. P. (2000) Communication: The royal pathway to patient-centred medicine. *Patient Education and Counselling*, 39, 1–3.

Berger, P. (1963) *Invitation to Sociology. A Humanistic Perspective*. New York, Anchor Books: Doubley & Company.

Berger, P. L. and Luckmann, T. (1966) *The Social Construction of Reality*. Garden City, New York: Anchor Books.

Berger, P. L. and Luckmann, T. (2002) The social construction of reality. In Calhoun, C., Gerteis, J., Moody, J., Pfaff, S. and Virk, I. (eds) *Contemporary Sociological Theory*. Oxford: Blackwell, 42–50.

Best, S. (2003) *A Beginner's Guide to Social Theory*. London: Sage.

Bhaskar R. (1989a) *The Possibility of Naturalism* (2nd edition). Brighton: Harvester Wheatsheaf.

Bhaskar, R. (1978) *A Realist Theory of Science*. Brighton: Harvester Wheatsheaf.

Bhaskar, R. (1986) *Scientific Realism and Human Emancipation*. London: Verso.

Bhaskar, R. (1989a) *The Possibility of Naturalism: A Philosophical Critique of the Contemporary Human Sciences*. Hemel Hempstead: Harvester Wheatsheaf.

Bhaskar, R. (1989b) *Reclaiming Reality*. London: Verso.

Bijker, W. E. (1995) *Of Bicycles, Bakelites and Bulbs: Towards a Theory of Sociotechnical Change*. Cambridge, MA: MIT Press.

Bijker, W. E., Hughes, T. P. and Pinch, T. (eds) ([1987] 1990) *The Social Construction of Technological Systems: New Directions in the Sociology and History of Technology*. Cambridge, MA: MIT Press.

Birke, L. (1999) *Feminism and the Biological Body*. New Brunswick, NJ: Rutgers University Press.

Birke, L. (2003) Shaping biology: Feminism and the idea of 'the biological'. In Williams, S. J., Birke, L. and Bendelow, G. A. (eds) *Debating Biology: Sociological Reflections on Health, Medicine and Society*. London: Routledge, 39–52.

Blackford, J. and Street, A. (2002) Cultural conflict: The impact of eastern feminism(s) on nurses caring for women of non-English speaking background. *Journal of Clinical Nursing*, 11(2), 664–671.

Blaxter, M. (2000) Medical sociology at the start of the new millennium. *Social Science and Medicine*, 51(8), 1139–1142.

Bloor, D. ([1976] 1991) *Knowledge and Social Imagery* (2nd edition). Chicago: Chicago University Press.

Blumer, H. (1954) What is wrong with social theory? *American Journal of Sociology*, 19 (February), 3–11.

Blumer, H. (2002) Symbolic interactionism. In Calhoun, C., Gerteis, J., Moody, J., Pfaff, S. and Virk, I. (eds) *Contemporary Sociological Theory*. Oxford: Blackwell, 66–77.

Boneham, M. A. and Sixsmith, J. A. (2006) The voices of older women in a disadvantaged community: Issues of health and social capital. *Social Science and Medicine*, 62(2), 269–279.

Boswell, J. (1998) *Life of Johnson*. Oxford: Oxford University Press.

Bourdieu, P. (1979) *Distinction: A Social Critique of the Judgement of Taste*. London: Routledge.

Bourdieu, P. (1986) The forms of capital. In Richardson, J. G. (ed.) *The Handbook of Theory and Research for the Sociology of Education*. New York: Greenwood Press, 241–258.

Bourret, P. (2005) BRCA patients and clinical collectives: New configurations of action in cancer genetics practices. *Social Studies of Science*, 35(1), 41–68.

Britten, N. (2001) Prescribing and the defense of clinical autonomy. *Sociology of Health and Illness*, 23(4), 478–496.

Brannen, J. (1988) Research note: The study of sensitive subjects. *The Sociological Review*, 36(1), 552–563.

Brown, N., Rappert, B. and Webster, A. (eds) (2000) *Contested Futures: A Sociology of Prospective Techno-Science*. Aldershot: Ashgate.

Brownlie, J. and Howson, A. (2005) Leaps of faith and MMR: An empirical study of trust. *Sociology*, 39(2), 221–239.

Brownlie, J. and Howson, A. (2006) Between the demands of truth and government: Health practitioners, trust and immunization work. *Social Science and Medicine*, 62(2), 433–443.

Burnstein, J. M., Yan, R., Weller, I. and Abramson, B. L. (2003) Management of congestive heart failure: A gender gap may still exist. Observations from a contemporary cohort. *BMC Cardiovascular Disorders*, 3(1), 1.

Burton, L. (1975) *The Family Life of Sick Children*. London: Routledge and Kegan Paul.

Bury, M. (1982) Chronic illness as biographical disruption. *Sociology of Health and Illness*, 4(3), 167–182.

Bury, M. (2001) Illness narratives: Fact or fiction? *Sociology of Health and Illness*, 23(3), 263–285.

Butler, J. (1990) *Gender Trouble: Feminism and the Subversion of Identity*. London: Routledge.

Byng, R., Norman, I. and Redfern, S. (2005) Using realistic evaluation to evaluate a practice-level intervention to improve primary healthcare for patients with long-term mental illness. *Evaluation*, 11(1), 69–93.

Calhoun, C., Gerteis, J., Moody, J., Pfaff, S., Schmidt, K. and Virk, I. (2002) *Classical Sociological Theory*. Oxford: Blackwell.

Callon, M. ([1987] 1990) Society in the making: The study of technology as a tool for sociological analysis. In Bijker, W. E., Hughes, T. P and Pinch, T. (eds) *The Social Construction of Technological Systems: New Directions in the Sociology and History of Technology*. Cambridge, MA: MIT Press, 83–110.

Campbell, C. (2000) Social capital and health: Contextualizing health promotion within local community networks. In Schuller, T., Baron, S. and Field, J. (eds) *Social Capital: Critical Perspectives*. Oxford: Oxford University Press, 182–196.

Carpiano, R. M. (2006) Toward a neighborhood resource-based theory of social capital for health: Can Bourdieu and sociology help? *Social Science and Medicine*, 62(1), 165–175.

Cartwright, A. and Anderson, R. (1981) *General Practice Revisited: A Second Study of Patients and their Doctors*. London: Tavistock.

Casiday, R., Cresswell, T., Wilson, D. and Panter-Brick, C. (2006) A survey of UK parental attitudes to the MMR vaccine and trust in medical authority. *Vaccine*, 24(2), 177–184.

Cattell, V. (2001) Poor people, poor places, and poor health: The mediating role of social networks and social capital. *Social Science and Medicine*, 52(10), 1501–1516.

Chadwick, E. (1842) *Report of an Enquiry into the Sanitary Conditions of the Labouring Population of Great Britain*. London: Poor Law Commission.

Charmaz, K. (1983) Loss of self: A fundamental form of suffering in the chronically ill. *Sociology of Health and Illness*, 5(2), 168–195.

Charmaz, K. (2000) Experiencing chronic illness. In Albrecht, G. L., Fitzpatrick, R. and Scrimshaw, S. C. (eds) *The Handbook of Social Studies in Health and Medicine*. London: Sage, 277–292.

Checkland, K. (2004) National service frameworks and UK general practitioners: Street level bureaucrats at work? *Sociology of Health and Illness*, 26(7), 951–976.

Cheek, J. and Porter, S. (1997) Reviewing Foucault: Possibilities and problems for nursing and heal care. *Nursing Inquiry*, 4(2), 108–119.

Chen, Y., Subramanian, S. V., Acevedo-Garcia, D., and Kawachi, I. (2005) Women's status and depressive symptoms: A multilevel analysis. *Social Science and Medicine*, 60(1), 49–60.

Chesler, P. (1972) *Women and Madness*. New York: Doubleday.

Churchill, W. (2005) The medical practice of the sexed body: Women, men, and disease in Britain, circa 1600–1740. *Social History of Medicine*, 18(1), 3–22.

Clarke, A. E., Mamo, L., Fishman, J. R., Shim, J. K. and Fosket, J. R. (2003) Biomedicalization: Technoscientific transformations of health, illness and US biomedicine. *American Sociological Review*, 68(2), 161–193.

Coalition for Improving Maternity Services (2007) The Coalition for Improving Maternity Services: Evidence basis for the ten steps of mother friendly care. *Journal of Perinatal Education*, 16(Suppl. 1), 1–93.

Coburn, D. (1993) State authority, medical dominance and the trends in the regulation of the health professions: The Ontario Case. *Social Science and Medicine*, 37(2), 129–138.

Cochrane, A. (1972) *Effectiveness and Efficiency: Random reflections on health services*. London: Nuffield Hospitals Trust.

Cohen, D., Farley, T. and Mason K. (2003) Why is poverty unhealthy? Social and physical mediators. *Social Science and Medicine*, 57(9), 1631–1641.

Coleman, J. S. (1988) Social capital in the creation of human capital. *American Journal of Sociology*, 94(s1), 95–120.

Collier, A. (1994) *Critical Realism*. London: Verso.

Conrad, P. (1992) Medicalization and social control. *Annual Review of Sociology*, 18 (August), 209–232.

Conrad, P. (1999) The mirage of genes. *Sociology of Health and Illness*, 21(2), 228–241.

Conrad, P. (2004a) The experience of illness. In Conrad, P. (ed.) *The Sociology of Health and Illness: Critical Perspectives* (7th edition). New York: Worth Publishers, 130–132.

Conrad, P. (2004b) The meaning of medication: Another look at compliance. In Conrad, P. (ed.) *The Sociology of Health and Illness: Critical Perspectives* (7th edition). New York: Worth Publishers, 150–162.

Conrad, P. and Angell, A. (2004) Homosexuality and remedicalization. *Society*, 41(5), 32–39.

Conrad, P. and Gabe, J. (eds) (1999) *Sociological Perspectives on the New Genetics*. Oxford: Blackwell.

Conrad, P. and Potter, D. (2000) From hyperactive children to ADHD adults: Observations on the expansion of medical categories. *Social Problems*, 47(4), 559–582.

Conrad, P. and Schneider, J. W. (1992) *Deviance and Medicalization: From Badness to Sickness*. Philadelphia: Temple University Press.

Cooper, H., Arber, S., Fee, L. and Ginn, J. (1999) *The Influence of Social Support and Social Capital on Health: A Review and Analysis of British Data*. London: Health Education Authority.

Coser, L. (ed.) (1965) *Georg Simmel*. Englewood Cliffs, NJ: Prentice Hall.

Coulter, A. and Fitzpatrick, R. (2000) The patient perspective regarding appropriate health care. In Albrecht, G. L., Fitzpatrick, R. and Scrimshaw, S. C. (eds) *The Handbook of Social Studies in Health and Medicine*. London: Sage, 454–464.

Courtnenay, W. H. (2000) Constructions of masculinity and their influence on men's well-being: A theory of gender and health. *Social Science and Medicine*, 50(10), 1385–1401.

Cox, S. M. and Starzomski, R. C. (2004) Genes and geneticization? The social construction of autosomal dominant polycystic kidney disease. *New Genetics and Society*, 23(2), 138–166.

Craig, G. M. and Scambler, G. (2006) Negotiating mothering against the odds: Gastrostomy tube feeding, stigma, governmentality and disabled children. *Social Science and Medicine*, 62(5), 1115–1125.

Crotty, M. (1996) *Phenomenology and Nursing Research*. Melbourne: Churchill Livingstone.

Crotty, M. (1998) *The Foundations of Social Research: Meaning and Perspective in the Research Process*. London: Sage.

Cunningham-Burley, S. and Boulton, M. (2000) The Social Context of the New Genetics. In Albrecht, G. L., Fitzpatrick, R. and Scrimshaw, S. C. (eds) *The Handbook of Social Studies in Health and Medicine*. London: Sage, 173–187.

Cunningham-Burley, S. and Kerr, A. (1999) Defining the 'social': Towards an understanding of scientific and medical discourses on the social aspects of the new human genetics. In Conrad, P. and Gabe, J. (eds) *Sociological Perspectives on the New Genetics*. Oxford: Blackwell, 149–170.

Curry, P. and O'Brien, M. (2006) The male heart and the female mind: A study in the gendering of antidepressants and cardiovascular drugs in advertisements in Irish medical publication. *Social Science and Medicine*, 62(8), 1970–1977.

Cwikel, J., Gramotnev, H. and Lee, C. (2006) Never-married childless women in Australia: Health and social circumstances in older age. *Social Science and Medicine*, 62(8), 1991–2001.

Dabral Datta, G., Subramanian, S. V., Colditz, G. A., Kawachi, I., Palmer, J. R. and Rosenberg, L. (2006) Individual, neighborhood, and state-level predictors of smoking among US Black women: A multilevel analysis. *Social Science and Medicine*, 63(4), 1034–1044.

Dalsgaard Reventlow, S., Hvas, L. and Malterud, K. (2006) Making the invisible body visible. Bone scans, osteoporosis and women's bodily experiences. *Social Science and Medicine*, 62(11), 2720–2731.

Davey Smith, G., Blane, D. and Bartley, M. (1994). Explanations for socio-economic differentials in mortality. *European Journal of Public Health*, 4, 131–144.

David, M. (2005) *Science in Society*. Basingstoke, Hampshire: Palgrave.

Davies, C. (1995) *Gender and the Professional Predicament in Nursing*. Buckingham: Open University Press.

Davis, K. (2007) Reclaiming women's bodies: Colonist trope or critical epistemology? *The Sociological Review*, 55(Suppl. 1), 50–64.

De Beauvoir, S. (1989 [1949/1957]) *The Second Sex*. Vintage: New York.

Delanty, G. (1999) *Social Theory in a Changing World: Conceptions of Modernity.* Polity Press: Cambridge.

Delanty, G. (2005) *Social Science Philosophical and Methodological Foundations* (2nd edition). Buckingham: Open University Press.

Di Cecco, R., Patel, U., and Upshur, R. (2002) Is there a clinically significant gender bias in post-myocardial infarction pharmacological management in the older (>60) population of a primary care practice? *BMC Family Practice.* 3(1), 8.

Diderichsen, F. (1995) Market reforms in health care and sustainability of the welfare state: Lessons from Sweden. *Health Policy,* 32(3), 141–153.

Dingley, C. and Roux, G. (2003) Inner strength in older Hispanic women with chronic illness. *Journal of Cultural Diversity,* 10(1), 11–22.

Dixon-Woods, M., Williams, S. J., Jackson, C. J., Akkad, A., Kenyon, S. and Habiba, M. (2006) Why do women consent to surgery, even when they do not want to? An interactionist and Bourdieusian analysis. *Social Science and Medicine,* 62(11), 2742–2753.

DoH (1997) The New National Health Service. London: Stationary office.

DoH (2006a) Department of Health. Good doctors, safer patients: Proposals to strengthen the system to assure and improve the performance of doctors and to protect the safety of patients. A report by the Chief Medical Officer Sir Liam Donaldson. London: DoH.

DoH (2006b) Department of Health. Medicines matters. London: DoH.

DoH (2007) Department of Health, Trust, assurance and safety – the regulation of health professionals. http://www.dh.gov.uk/en/Publicationsandstatistics/Publications/PublicationsPolicyAndGuidance/DH_065946, last accessed April 2007.

DoHC (2007) Medical Practitioners Bill. Dublin: Department of Health and Children.

Donelan, K., Blendon, R. J., Schoen, C., Davis, K. and Binns, K. (1999) The cost of health system change: Public discontent in five nations. *Health Affairs,* 18, 206–216.

Doyal, L. and Anderson, J. (2005) 'My fear is to fall in love again...' How HIV-positive African women survive in London. *Social Science and Medicine,* 60(8), 1729–1738.

Doyal, L. and Gough, I. (1991) *A Theory of Human Need.* London: Macmillan.

Doyal, L. with Pennell, I. (1979) *The Political Economy of Health.* London: Pluto Press.

du Pré (2002) Accomplishing the impossible: Talking about body and soul and mind during a medical visit. *Health Communication,* 14(1), 1–21.

Dubos, R. (1959) *Mirage of Health.* New York: Harper Row.

Dunnell, K. and Cartwright, A. (1972) *Medicine Takers, Prescribers and Hoarders.* London: Routledge and Kegan Paul.

Durkheim, É. ([1897] 1951) *Suicide.* New York: Free Press.

Durkheim, É. ([1893] 1964) *The Division of Labour in Society.* New York: Free Press.

Durkheim, E. ([1895] 1982) What is a Social Fact? In *The Rules of the Sociological Method* (Edited by Steven Lukes; Translated by W. D. Halls). New York: Free Press, 50–59.

Eagleton, T. (1991) *Ideology: An Introduction*. London: Verso.

Edge, D. and Rogers, A. (2005) Dealing with it: Black Caribbean women's response to adversity and psychological distress associated with pregnancy, childbirth, and early motherhood. *Social Science and Medicine*, 61(1), 15–25.

Ehrenreich, B. and English, D. (1974) *Complaints and Disorders. The Sexual Politics of Sickness*. London: Compendium.

Ehrenreich, B. (1976) What is socialist feminism? *Working Papers on Socialism and Feminism*. Chicago: New American Movement.

El-Nemer, A., Downe, S. and Small, N. (2006) 'She would help me from the heart': An ethnography of Egyptian women in labour. *Social Science and Medicine*, 62(1), 81–92.

Elston, M. A. (1991) The politics of professional power: Medicine in a changing health service. In Gabe, J., Calnan, M. and Bury, M. (eds) *The Sociology of the Health Service*. London: Routledge, 58–88.

Emslie, C., Hunt, K. and Watt, G. (2003) A chip off the old block? Lay understandings of inheritance among men and women in mid-life. *Public Understanding of Science*, 12(1), 47–65.

Engels, F. ([1886] 1987) *The Condition of the Working Classes in England*. New York: Penguin books. English translation first published in 1886 in New York by Victor Kiernan.

Evans, J. (1995) *Feminist Theory Today: An Introduction to Second-Wave Feminism*. London: Sage.

Evans, M. (2003) *Gender and Social Theory*. Buckingham: Open University Press.

Fassin, D. (2000). Qualifier les inégalites. In Leclerc, A., Fassin, D., Grandjean, H., Kaminski, M. and Lang, T. (eds) *Les Inégalites socials de sante*. Paris: INSERM/La Découverte, 124–144.

Fausto-Sterling, A. (2003) The problem with sex/gender and nature/nature. In Simon, J., Williams, S. J., Birke, L. and Bendelow, G. A. (eds) *Debating Biology: Sociological Reflections on Health, Medicine and Society*. London: Routledge, 123–132.

Ferguson, H. (2001) Phenomenology and social theory. In Ritzer, G. and Smart, B. (eds) *Handbook of Social Theory*. London: Sage, 232–248.

Ferrell, B. (2005) Ethical perspectives on pain and suffering. *Pain Management Nursing*, 6(3), 83–90.

Finch, J. (1984) 'It's great to have someone to talk to': The ethics and politics of interviewing women. In Bell, C. and Roberts, H. (eds) *Social Researching: Politics, Problems, Practice*. London: Routledge and Kegan Paul, 70–87.

Firestone, S. (1971) *The Dialectic of Sex*. London: Jonathan Cape.

Fisher, C., Hauck, Y. and Fenwick, J., (2006) How social context impacts on women's fears of childbirth: A Western Australia example. *Social Science and Medicine*, 63(1), 64–75.

Flax, J. (1990) Postmodernism and gender relations in feminist theory. In Nicholson, L. (ed.), *Feminism/Postmodernism*. London: Routledge, 39–62.

Fleck, L. ([1935] 1979) *Genesis and Development of a Scientific Fact* (Translated by F. Bradley, T. J. Trenn and R. K. Merton). Chicago: University of Chicago Press.

Flynn, R. (2002) Clinical governance and governmentality. *Health, Risk and Society*, 4(2), 155–173.

Foucault, M. ([1973] 1976) *The Birth of the Clinic: An Archaeology of Medical Perception*. London: Tavistock.

Foucault, M. (1973) *The Birth of the Clinic: An Archeology of Medical Perception* (Translated by A. M. Sheridan Smith). London: Tavistock.

Foucault, M. (1979) *Discipline and Punish: The Birth of the Prison*. London: Penguin.

Foucault, M. (1980) Body/power. In Gordon, C. (ed.) *Power/Knowledge: Selected Interviews and Other Writings by Michel Foucault, 1972–1977*. New York: Pantheon, 55–63.

Foucault, M. (1984a) *The Will to Knowledge: The History of Sexuality Volume 1*. London: Penguin.

Foucault, M. (1984b) Truth and Power. In Rabinow, P. (ed.) *The Foucault Reader*. New York: Pantheon, 51–75.

Foucault, M. (1985) *The Use of Pleasure: The History of Sexuality Volume 2*. London: Penguin.

Foucault, M. (1986) *The Care of the Self: The History of Sexuality Volume 3*. London: Penguin.

Foucault, M. (1988) Technologies of the self. In Martin, L. H., Gutman, H. and Hutton, P. H. (eds) *Technologies of the Self: A Seminar with Michel Foucault*. Amherst, MA: University of Massachusetts Press, 16–49.

Foucault, M. (1991) Governmentality. In Burchell, G., Gordon, C. and Miller, P. (eds) *The Foucault Effect: Studies in Governmentality*. London: Harvester Wheatsheaf, 87–104.

Fox Keller, E. (2000) *The Century of the Gene*. Cambridge, MA: Harvard University Press.

Fox, N. J. (1997) Is there life after Foucault? Texts, frames and differends. In Petersen, A. and Bunton, R. (eds) *Foucault, Health and Medicine*. London and New York: Routledge, 31–50.

Fraser, N. and Nicholson, L. J. (1988) Social criticism without philosophy: An encounter between feminism and postmodernism. *Communication*, 10(3), 345–366.

Freidson, E. (1970a) *The Profession of Medicine: A Study of the Applied Sociology of Knowledge*. New York: Dodd Mead.

Freidson, E. (1970b) *Professional Dominance: The Social Structure of Medical Care*. Chicago: Aldine.

Freidson, E. (1974) Dominant professions, bureaucracy and client services. In Hasenfeld, Y. and English, R. A. (eds) *Human Service Organizations*. Ann Arbor: University of Michigan Press.

Freidson, E. (1986) *Professional Powers: A Study of the Institutionalization of Formal Knowledge*. Chicago: University of Chicago Press.

Freidson, E. (1994). *Professionalism Reborn*. Cambridge: Polity Press.

Freund, P. E. S. (1990) The expressive body: A common ground for the sociology of emotions and health and illness. *Sociology of Health and Illness*, 12(4), 452–477.

Gamarnikow, E. (1978) Sexual divisions of labour: The case of nursing. In Kuhn, A. and Wolpe, A. M. (eds) *Feminism and Materialism*, London: Routledge and Kegan Paul, 96–123.

Garfinkel, H. (1967) *Studies in Ethnomethodology*. Englewood Cliffs, NJ: Prentice-Hall.

Garfinkel, H. (1991) Respecification: Evidence for locally produced, naturally accountable phenomena of order, logic, reason, meaning, method, etc. in and as of the essential haecceity of immortal ordinary society (1): An announcement of studies. In Button G. (ed.) *Ethnomethodology and the Human Sciences*. Cambridge: Cambridge University Press, 10–19.

Giddens, A. (1976) *New Rules of Sociological Method*. London: Hutchinson.

Gilbert, T. (2005) Trust and managerialism: Exploring discourses of care. *Journal of Advanced Nursing*, 52(4), 454–463.

Gilligan, C. (1982) *In a Different Voice: Psychological Theory and Women's Development*. Cambridge, MA: Harvard University Press.

Glaser, B. and Strauss, A. L. ([1967] 1999) *The Discovery of Grounded Theory: Strategies for Qualitative Research*. New York: Aldine de Gruyter.

Glendinning, C. (1983) *Unshared Care: Parents and their Disabled Children*. London: Routledge and Kegan Paul.

Goffman, E. (1963) *Stigma: Notes on the Management of Spoiled Identity*. Englewood Cliffs, NJ: Prentice-Hall.

Goffman, E. ([1956] 1969) *The Presentation of Self in Everyday Life*. London: Penguin Press.

Goffman, E. ([1961] 1998) Asylums. In Mackay, L., Soothill, K. and Melia, K. (eds) *Classic Texts in Health Care*. Oxford: Butterworth Heinemann, 100–104.

Gordon, C. (1991) Governmental Rationality: An Introduction. In Burchell, G., Gordon, C. and Miller, P. (eds) *The Foucault Effect: Studies in Governmentality*. London: Harvester Wheatsheaf, 1–52.

Gough, B. and Conner, M. T. (2006) Barriers to healthy eating amongst men: A qualitative analysis. *Social Science and Medicine*, 62(2), 387–395.

Graham, H. (1983) Do her answers fit his questions? Women and the survey method. In Gamarnikow, E., Morgan, D., Purvis, J., Taylorson, D. (eds) *The Public and the Private*. London: Heinemann Educational Books, 132–146.

Graham, H. (1984) Surveying through stories. In Bell, C. and Roberts, H. (eds) *Social Researching: Politics, Problems, Practice*. London: Routledge and Kegan Paul, 104–124.

Graham, H. (2002). Building an inter-disciplinary science of health inequalities: The example of life-course research. *Social Science and Medicine*, 55(11), 2006–2016.

Grann, V., Troxel, A. B., Zojwalla, N., Hershman, D., Glied, S. A. and Jacobson, J. S. (2006) Regional and racial disparities in breast cancer-specific mortality. *Social Science and Medicine*, 62, 337–347.

Green, S. and Higgins, J. (eds) *Glossary. Cochrane Handbook for Systematic Reviews of Interventions 4.2.5 [updated May 2005].* http://www.cochrane.org/resources/handbook/accessed May 3, 2008.

Greenhalgh, T., Glenn, R., Bate, P., Kyriakidou, O., Macfarlane, F. and Peacock, R. (2004) *How to Spread Good Ideas: A Systematic Review of the Literature on Diffusion, Dissemination and Sustainability of Innovations in Health Service Delivery and Organization.* London: NCCSDO.

Hafferty, F. and Light, D. (1995) Professional dynamics and the changing nature of medical work, *Journal of Health and Social Behavior* (Extra), 132–153.

Hafferty, F. W. and McKinlay, J. B. (1993) *The Changing Medical Profession: An International Perspective.* Oxford: Oxford University Press.

Hales, L., Lohan, M. and Jordan, J. (2007) New Doctor-Nurse Partnerships in Practice? The case of Supplementary Prescribing. Paper Presented to BSA medical Sociology Group Annual Conference, Liverpool. September 2007.

Hall, P., Brockington, I., Levings, J. and Hughes, G. H. (1993) Comparisons of responses to the mentally ill in two communities. *British Journal of Psychiatry,* 162, 99–108.

Haraway, D. (1999) The visual speculum in the New World Order. In Clarke, A. E. and Olesen, V. L. (eds) *Revisioning Women, Health, and Healing.* New York: Routledge, 49–96.

Harrison, S. (2002) New labour, modernisation and the medical labour process. *Journal of Social Policy,* 31(3), 465–485.

Harrison, S. and Politt, C. (1994) *Controlling Health Professionals: The Future of Work and Organization in the NHS.* Buckingham: Open University Press.

Harste, G. and Mortensen, N. (2000) Social interaction theories. In Andersen, H. and Bo Kaspersen, L. (eds) *Classical and Modern Social Theory.* Oxford: Blackwell, 176–196.

Hartley, H. (2002) The system of alignments challenging physician professional dominance: An elaborated theory of countervailing powers. *Sociology of Health and Illness,* 24(2), 178–207.

Haug, M. (1973) Deprofessionalization: An alternative hypothesis for the future. *Sociological Review Monograph,* 2, 195–211.

Hawe, P. and Shiell, A. (2000) Social capital and health promotion: A review. *Social Science and Medicine,* 51(6), 871–885.

Heymenn, J., Hertzman, C., Barer, M. L. and Evans, R. G. (eds) (2006) *Healthier Societies: From Analysis to Action.* Oxford: Oxford University Press.

Hedgecoe, A. (2006) Pharmacogenetics as alien science: Alzheimer's disease, core sets and expectations. *Social Studies of Science,* 36(5), 723–752.

Hedgecoe, A. and Martin, P. (2003) The drugs don't work: Expectations and the shaping of pharmacogenetics. *Social Studies of Science,* 33(3), 327–364.

Hedgecoe, A. M. (2002) Reinventing diabetes: Classification, division and the geneticization of disease. *New Genetics and Society,* 21(1), 7–27.

Hekman, S. (1990) *Gender and Knowledge: Elements of a Postmodern Feminism* Cambridge: Polity Press.

Heidegger, M. ([1927] 1982) *The Basic Problems of Phenomenology* (Translated by Albert Hofstadter). Bloomington: Indiana University Press.

Hemmings, C. (2005) Telling feminist stories. *Feminist Theory*, 6(2), 115–139.

Herman, R. J. (1993) Return to sender: Reintegrative stigma-management strategies of ex-psychiatric patients. *Journal of Contemporary Ethnography*, 22(3), 295–330.

Higgins, J. P. T. and Green, S. (eds) (2008) The Cochrane collaboration, *Cochrane Handbook for Systematic Reviews of Interventions*, http://www.cochrane-handbook.org, Version 5.0.1 (updated September 2008).

Higgs, P. (1989) Risk, governmentality and the reconceptualisation of citizenship. In Higgs, P. and. Scambler, G (eds) *Modernity, Medicine and Health*. London: Routledge, 176–197.

Hill Collins, P. (2001) Defining Black feminist thought. In Essed, P. and Goldberg, A. T. (eds) *Race Critical Theories: Text and Context*. Malden, Mass: Blackwell Publishing, 152–175.

Hobson-West, P. (2007) Trusting blindly can be the biggest risk of all: Organized resistance to childhood vaccination in the UK. *Sociology of Health and Illness*, 29(2), 198–215.

Hochschild, A. R. (1983) *The Managed Heart: Commercialization of Human Feeling*. Berkeley: University of California Press.

Holmwood, J. (1995) Feminism and epistemology: What kind of successor science? *Sociology*, 29(3), 411–428.

Holton, R. and Turner, B. (1989) *Max Weber on Economy and Society*. London: Routledge.

Howson, A. (2005) *Embodying Gender*. London: Sage.

Hughes, B. and Patterson, K. (1997) The social model of disability and the disappearing body: A sociology of impairment. *Disability and Society*, 12(3), 325–340.

Hughes, D. (1988) When nurse knows best: Some aspects of nurse-doctor interaction in a casualty department. *Sociology of Health and Illness*, 10(1), 1–22.

Hume, D. ([1739–1740] 1969) *A Treatise on Human Nature*. Harmondsworth: Penguin.

Humm, M. (1995) *The Dictionary of Feminist Theory* (2nd edition). London: Prentice Hall.

Hunt, K. and Annandale, E. (1999) Relocating gender and morbidity: Examining men's and women's health in contemporary Western societies. Introduction to Special Issue on Gender and Health. *Social Science and Medicine*, 48(1), 1–5.

Hunter, D. J. (1994) From tribalism to corporatism: The managerial challenge to medical dominance. In Gabe, J., Kelleher, D. and Williams, G. (eds) *Challenging Medicine*. London: Routledge, 1–22.

Husserl, E. ([1913] 1982) *Ideas Pertaining to a Pure Phenomenology and to a Phenomenological Philosophy* (Translated by F. Kersten). The Hague: Nijhoff.

Hutton, P. H. (1988) Foucault, Freud, and the technologies of the self. In Martin, L. H., Gutman, H. and Hutton, P. H. (eds) *Technologies of the Self: Seminar with Michel Foucault*. Amherst, MA: University of Massachusetts Press, 121–144.

Huynh, M., Parker, J. D., Harper, S., Pamuk, E. and Schoendorf, K. C. (2005) Contextual effect of income inequality on birth outcomes. *International Journal of Epidemiology*, 34(4), 888–895.

Hyde, A., Lohan, M. and McDonnell, O. (2004) *Sociology for Health Professionals in Ireland*. Dublin: Institute of Public Administration.

Inhorn, M. C. and Whittle, K. L. (2001) Feminism meets the 'new' epidemiologies: Towards an appraisal of antifeminist biases in epidemiological research on women's health. *Social Science and Medicine*, 53(5), 553–567.

International Council for Nurses (2004) *Implementing Nurse Prescribing*. Geneva: ICN.

James, N. (1989) Emotional labour: Skill and work in the social regulation of feelings. *Sociological Review*, 37(1), 15–41.

James, V. and Gabe, J. (eds) (1996) *Health and the Sociology of Emotions*. Oxford: Blackwell Publishers.

Kant, I. ([1781] 1907) *Critique of Pure Reason*. New York: Macmillan.

Kaplan, J. M. (2000) *The Limits and Lies of Human Genetic Research: Dangers for Social Policy*. New York and London: Routledge.

Kawachi, I. and Kennedy, B. P. (1999) Income inequality and health: Pathways and mechanisms. *Health Services Research*, 34(1), 215–227.

Kawachi, I., Kennedy, B. P. and Glass, R. (1999a) Social capital and self-rated health: A contextual analysis. *American Journal of Public Health*, 89(8), 1187–1193.

Kawachi, I., Kennedy, B. P. and Wilkinson, R. G. (eds) (1999b). *The Society and Population Health Reader: Vol. 1 Income Inequality and Health*. New York: New Press.

Kawachi, I., Kennedy, B. P., Lochner, K. and Prothrow-Stith, D. (1997) Social capital, income inequality, and mortality. *American Journal of Public Health*, 87(9), 1491–1498.

Kawachi, I., Subramanian, S. V. and Almeida-Filho, N. (2002) A glossary for health inequalities. *Journal of Epidemiology and Community Health*, 56(9), 647–652.

Kazi, M. (2003a) *Realist Evaluation in Practice*. London: Sage.

Kazi, M. (2003b) Realist evaluation for practice. *British Journal of Social Work*, 33(6), 803–818.

Kegan Gardiner, J. (2005) Men masculinities and feminist theory. In Kimmel, M. S., Hearn, J. and Connell, R. W. (eds) *Handbook of Studies on Men and Masculinities*. London: Sage, 35–50.

Kempner, J. (2006) Gendering the migraine market: Do representations of illness matter? *Social Science and Medicine*, 63(8), 1986–1997.

Kendall, C., Afable-Munsuz, A., Speizer, I., Avery, A., Schmidt, N. and Santelli, J. (2005) Understanding pregnancy in a population of inner-city women in New Orleans – results of qualitative research. *Social Science and Medicine*, 60(2), 297–311.

Kent, J. (2000) *Social Perspectives on Pregnancy and Childbirth for Midwives, Nurses and the Caring Professions*. Buckingham: Open University Press.

Kerr, A. and Cunningham-Burley, S. (2000) On ambivalence and risk: Reflexive modernity and the new human genetics. *Sociology*, 34(2), 283–304.

Klein, R. (1990) The state and the profession: The politics of the double bed. *British Medical Journal*, 301(6754), 700–702.

Kleinman, A. (1988) *The Illness Narratives: Suffering, Health and the Human Condition*. New York: Basic Books.

Kleinman, A. and Seeman, D. (2000) Personal experience of illness. In Albrecht, G. L., Fitzpatrick, R. and Scrimshaw, S. C. (eds) *The Handbook of Social Studies in Health and Medicine*. London: Sage, 230–242.

Knorr-Cetina, K. D. (1983) The ethnographic study of scientific work: Towards a constructivist interpretation of science. In Knorr-Cetina, K. D. and Mulkay, M. (eds) *Science Observed: Perspectives on the Social Study of Science*. London: Sage, 115–140.

Knorr-Cetina, K. D. and Mulkay, M. (1983) Introduction: Emerging principles in the social studies of science. In Knorr-Cetina, K. D. and Mulkay, M. (eds) *Science Observed: Perspectives on the Social Study of Science*. London: Sage, 1–18.

Krimsky, S. (2001) Journal policies on conflict of interest: If this is therapy, what's the disease? *Psychotherapy and Psychosomatics*, 70, 115–117.

Krimsky, S., Rothenberg, L. S., Stott, P. and Kyke, G. (1999) Scientific journals and their authors' financial interests: A pilot study. In Caulfield, T. A. and Williams-Jones, B. (eds) *The Commercialization of Genetic Research: Ethical, Legal, and Policy Issues*. New York: Kluwer Academic/Plenum Publishers, 101–110.

Kritzer, H. M. (1999) The professions are dead, long live the professions: Legal practice in a post-professional world, *Law and Society Review*, 33(3), 713–759.

Kruks, S. (2001) *Retrieving Experience: Subjectivity and Recognition in Feminist Politics*. London: Cornell University Press.

Kuhlmann, K. and Babitsch, B. (2002) Bodies, health, gender – bridging feminist theories and women's health. *Women's Studies International Forum*, 25(4), 433–442.

Kuhn, T. S. (1962) *The Structure of Scientific Revolutions*. Chicago: University of Chicago Press.

Kunitz, S. J. (2004) Social capital and health. *British Medical Bulletin*, 69, 61–73.

Laqueur, T. (1990) *Making Sex: Body and Gender from the Greeks to Freud*. Cambridge, MA: Harvard University Press.

Lash, S. and Urry, J. (1994) *Economics of Signs and Space*. London: Sage.

Latour, B. (1983) Give me a laboratory and I will raise the world. In Knorr-Cetina, K. and Mulkay, M. (eds) *Science Observed: Perspective on the Social Study of Science*. London: Sage, 141–170.

Latour, B. (1987) *Science in Action: How to Follow Scientists and Engineers Through Society*. Cambridge, MA: Harvard University Press.

Latour, B. and Woolgar, S. ([1979] 1986) *Laboratory Life: The Construction of Scientific Facts* (2nd edition). Princeton, NJ: Princeton University Press.

Law, J. ([1987] 1990) Technology and heterogeneous engineering: The case of Portuguese expansion. In Bijker, W. E., Hughes, T. P. and Pinch, T. (eds) *The Social Construction of Technological Systems: New Directions in the Sociology and History of Technology*. Cambridge, MA: MIT Press, 111–134.

Lawrence, S. C. and Bendixen, K. (1992) His and hers: Male and female anatomy in anatomy texts for US medical students, 1890–1989. *Social Science and Medicine*, 35(7), 925–934.

Lawson, T. (1997) *Economics and Reality*. London: Routledge.

Lawton, J. (2003) Lay experiences of health and illness: Past research and future agendas. *Sociology of Health and Illness*, 25(1), 23–40.

Lawton, R. (1998) Not working to rule: Understanding procedural violations at work. *Safety Science*, 28(2), 77–95.

Lawton, R. and Parker, D. (1999) Procedures and the professional: The case of the British NHS *Social Science and Medicine*, 48(3), 353–361.

Layder, D. (1994) *Understanding Social Theory*. London: Sage.

Lee, J. D. and Craft, E. A. (2002) Protecting one's self from a stigmatized diseases… Once one has it. *Deviant Behaviour*, 23(3), 267–299.

Lehtinen, E. (2005) Information, understanding and the benign order of everyday life in genetic counseling. *Sociology of Health and Illness*, 27(5), 575–601.

Leicht, K., Fennell, M. and Witkowski, K. (1995) The effects of hospital characteristics and radical organizational change on the relative standing of health care professions. *Journal of Health and Social Behavior*, 36 (June), 151–167.

Letherby, G. (2003) *Feminist Research in Theory and Practice*. McGraw Hill.

Lewis, J. and Meredith, B. (1988). *Daughters Who Care: Daughters Caring for Their Mothers at Home*. London: Routledge.

Lewontin, R. C. (1991) *Biology as Ideology: The Doctrine of DNA*. New York: Harper Perennial.

Liamputtong, P. (2005) Birth and social class: Northern Thai women's experiences of caesarean and vaginal birth. *Sociology of Health and Illness*, 27(2), 243–270.

Light, D. (1993) Countervailing power: The changing character of the medical profession in the United States. In Hafferty, F. and McKinlay, J. (eds) *The Changing Medical Profession: An International Perspective*. New York: Oxford University Press, 69–80.

Light, D. (2000) The medical profession and organizational change: From professional dominance to countervailing power. In Bird, C., Conrad, P. and Fremont, A. (eds) *Handbook of Medical Sociology* (5th edition). London: Prentice Hall, 201–216.

Lillrank, A. (2003) Back pain and the resolution of diagnostic uncertainty in illness narratives. *Social Science and Medicine*, 57(6), 1045–1054.

Lippman, A. (1991) Prenatal genetic testing and screening: Constructing needs and reinforcing inequalities. *American Journal of Law and Medicine*, 17(1/2), 15–50.

Lippman, A. (1998) The Politics of health: Genetization versus health promotion. In S. Shervin (ed.) *The Politics of Women's Health: Exploring Agency and Autonomy*. Philadelphia: Temple University Press, 64–82.

Locock, L. and Alexander, J. (2006) 'Just a bystander'? Men's place in the process of fetal screening and diagnosis. *Social Science and Medicine*, 62(6), 1349–1359.

Lohan, M. (2000) Constructive tensions in feminist technology studies. *Social Studies of Science*, 30(6), 895–916.

Lohan, M. (2007) How might we understand men's health better? Integrating explanations from critical studies on men and inequalities in health. *Social Science and Medicine*, 65(3), 493–504.

Lopez, K. A. and Willis, D. G. (2004) Descriptive versus interpretative phenomenology: Their contribution to nursing knowledge. *Qualitative Health Research*, 14(5), 726–735.

Lorber, J. (1997) *Gender and the Social Construction of Illness*. London: Sage.

Lupton, D. (1995) *The Imperative of Health: Public Health and the Regulated Body*. London: Sage.

Lupton, D. (1997) Consumerism, reflexivity and the medical encounter. *Social Science and Medicine*, 45(3), 373–381.

Lupton, D. (1997) Foucault and the medicalization critique. In Petersen, A. and Bunton, R. (eds) *Foucault, Health and Medicine*. London and New York: Routledge, 94–110.

Lupton, D. (2003) *Medicine as Culture: Illness, Disease and the Body in Western Societies* (2nd edition). London: Sage.

Lynch, J., Davey-Smith, G., Harper, S., Hillemeier, M., Ross, N., Kaplan, G. A. and Wolfson, M. (2004). Is income inequality a determinant of population health? Part 1. A systematic review. *The Milbank Quarterly*, 82(1), 5–99.

Lynch, J. W., Davey-Smith, G., Hillemeier, M., Shaw, M., Raghunathan, T. and Kaplan, G. (2001). Income inequality, the psychosocial environment and health: Comparisons of wealthy nations. *Lancet*, 358(9277), 194–200.

Lynch, J. W., Kaplan, G. A. and Salonen, J. T. (1997) Why do poor people behave poorly? Variation in adult health behaviours and psychosocial characteristics by stages of socioeconomic life course. *Social Science and Medicine*, 44(6), 809–819.

Lyndon, N. (1992) *No More Sex War. The Failures of Feminism*. London: Sinclair-Stevenson.

Macintyre, S. (1977) *Single and Pregnant*. London: Croom Helm.

Macintyre, S. (1991) Who wants babies? The social construction of instincts. In Leonard, D. and Allen, S. (eds) *Sexual Divisions Revisited*. London: Macmillan in association with the BSA.

Macintyre, S. (1997). The Black Report and beyond what are the issues? *Social Science and Medicine*, 44(6), 723–745.

Macintyre, S., Hunt, K. and Sweeting, H. ([1996] 2004) Gender differences in health: Are things really as they seem? In Bury, M. and Jonathan, G. (eds) *The Sociology of Health and Illness: A Reader*. London: Routledge, 161–171.

Macintyre, S., MacIver, S. and Sooman, A. (1993) Area, class and health: Should we be focusing on places or people? *Journal of Social Policy*, 22(2), 213–234.

MacKenzie, C. and Stoljar, N. (eds) (2000) *Relational Autonomy: Feminist Perspectives on Autonomy, Agency and the Social Self*. Oxford: Oxford University Press.

Macleod, J. and Davey Smith, G. (2003). Psychosocial factors and public health: A suitable case for treatment? *Journal of Epidemiology and Community Health,* 57, 565–570.

Madoo Lengermann, P. and Niebrugge-Brantley, J. (2003) Contemporary feminist theory. In Ritzer, G. and Goodman, D. J. (eds) *Sociological Theory.* New York: McGraw-Hill, 436–479.

Manderson, L., Markovic, M. and Quinn, M. (2005) 'Like roulette': Australian women's explanations of gynaecological cancers. *Social Science and Medicine,* 61(2), 323–332.

Mannheim, K. (1936) *Ideology and Utopia.* New York: Harcourt, Brace & company.

Manning, P. (1992) *Erving Goffman and Modern Sociology.* Cambridge: Polity Press.

Marmot, M. (2005) Social determinants of health inequalities. *Lancet,* 365(9464), 1099–1104.

Marmot, M. G. and Wilkinson, R. G. (2001) Psychosocial and material pathways in the relation between income and health: A response to Lynch *et al. British Medical Journal,* 322(7296), 1233–1236.

Martin, E. (2001) *The Woman in the Body: A Cultural Analysis of Reproduction.* Boston: Beacon Press.

Martin, P. (1999) Genes as drugs: The social shaping of gene therapy and the reconstruction of genetic disease. *Sociology of Health and Illness,* 21(5), 517–538.

Martin, P. (2001) Genetic governance: The risks, oversight and regulation of genetic databases in the UK. *New Genetics and Society,* 20(2), 157–183.

Martin, P. and Kaye, J. (2000) The use of large biological sample collections in genetics research: Issues for public policy. *New Genetics and Society,* 19(2), 165–191.

Martínez, R. G. (2005) 'What's wrong with me?': Cervical cancer in Venezuela – living in the borderlands of health, disease, and illness. *Social Science and Medicine,* 61(4), 797–808.

Marx, K. (1942) Wage, labour and capital. In *Selected Works Vol.1.* London: Lawrence and Wishart.

Marx, K. ([1852] 1954) *The Eighteenth Brumaire of Louis Bonaparte.* Moscow: Progress Publishers.

Marx, K. ([1857–1858] 1973a) *Grundrisse.* Harmondsworth: Penguin.

Marx, K. ([1852] 1973b) The Eighteenth Brumaire of Louis Bonaparte. In Marx, K. *Surveys from Exile.* Harmondsworth: Penguin.

Marx, K. ([1888] 1974) Theses on Feuerbach in Marx, K. and Engels, F. *The German Ideology.* London: Lawrence and Wishart.

Mathews, S., Manor, O. and Power, C. (1999) Social inequalities in health: Are there gender differences? *Social Science and Medicine,* 48(1), 49–60.

May, C., Rapley, T., Moreira, T., Finch, T. and Heaven, B. (2006) Technogovernance: Evidence, subjectivity, and the clinical encounter in primary care medicine. *Social Science and Medicine,* 62(4), 1022–1030.

Maynard, D. W. (2003) *Bad news, Good News: Conversational Order in Everyday Talk and Clinical Settings.* Chicago: The University of Chicago Press.

Mazhindu, D. and Brownsell, M. (2003) Piecemeal policy may stop nurse prescribers fulfilling their potential. *British Journal of Community Nursing*, 8(6), 253–255.

McCourt, C. (2006) Supporting choice and control? Communication and interaction between midwives and women at the antenatal booking visit. *Social Science and Medicine*, 62(6), 1307–1318.

McCoy, L. (2005) HIV-positive patients and the doctor-patient relationship: Perspectives from the margins. *Qualitative Health Research*, 15(6), 791–806.

McDowell, M. (1993) Measuring women's occupational mortality. *Population Trends*, 34, 25–29.

McEvoy, P. and Richards, D. (2003) Critical realism: A way forward for evaluation research in nursing? *Journal of Advanced Nursing*, 43(4), 411–420.

McEvoy, P. and Richards, D. (2006) A critical realist rationale for using a combination of quantitative and qualitative methods. *Journal of Research in Nursing*, 11(1), 66–78.

McKinlay, J. B. and Arches, J. (1985) Towards the proletarianization of physicians. *International Journal of Health Services*, 15(2), 161–195.

McKinlay, J. B. and Marceau, L. D. (2002) The end of the golden age of doctoring. *International Journal of Health Services*, 32(2), 379–416.

McKinlay, J. B. and Stoeckle, J. D. (1988) Corporatization and the social transformation of doctoring. *International Journal of Health Services*, 18(2), 191–205.

McLennan, G. (1995) Feminism, epistemology, and postmodernism: Reflections on current ambivalence. *Sociology*, 29(2) 391–409.

McMunn, A., Bartley, M. and Kuh, D. (2006) Women's health in mid-life: Life course social roles and agency as quality. *Social Science and Medicine*, 63(6), 1561–1572.

McNamara, M. S. (2005) Knowing and doing phenomenology: The implications of the critique of 'nursing phenomenology' for a phenomenological inquiry: A discussion paper. *International Journal of Nursing Studies*, 42(6), 695–704.

Mead, N. and Bower, P. (2000) Patient-centredness: A conceptual framework and review of the empirical literature. *Social Science and Medicine*, 51(7), 1087–1110.

Medical Research Council (2000) *Framework for Development and Evaluation RCTs for Complex Interventions to Improve Health*. London: MRC.

Melia, K. (1987) *Learning and Working: The Occupational Socialization of Nurses*. London: Tavistock.

Merton, R. K. (1968) *Social Theory and Social Structure, Enlarged Edition*. New York: The Free Press.

Merton, R. K. (1973) *The Sociology of Science: Theoretical and Empirical Investigations*. Chicago: University of Chicago Press.

Millett, K. (1977) *Sexual Politics*. London: Virago.

Mishler, E. G. (1984) *The Discourse of Medicine: Dialectics of Medical Interviews*. Norwood, NJ: Ablex.

Møldrup, C. (2002) When pharmacogenomics goes public. *New Genetics and Society*, 21(1), 29–37.

Moore, S., Shiell, A., Hawe, P. and Haines, V. A. (2005) The privileging of communitarian ideas: Citation practices and the translation of social capital into public health research. *American Journal of Public Health*, 95(8), 1330–1337.

Moran, M. (1999) *Governing the Health Care State: A Comparative Study of the United Kingdom, and the United States and Germany.* Manchester: Manchester University Press.

Morrison, K. (2006) *Marx, Durkheim and Weber Formations of Modern Social Thought* (2nd edition). London: Sage.

Moulding, N. (2006) Disciplining the feminine: The reproduction of gender contradictions in the mental health care of women with eating disorders. *Social Science and Medicine*, 62(4), 793–804.

Muntaner, C. and Lynch, J. (1999) Income inequality, social cohesion, and class relations: A critique of Wilkinson's neo-Durkheimian research program. *International Journal of Health Services*, 29(1), 59–81.

Murphy-Lawless, J. (1998) *Reading Birth and Death: A History of Obstetric Practice.* Cork: Cork University Press.

Nancarrow, S. A. and Borthwick, A. M. (2005) Dynamic professional boundaries in the healthcare workforce. *Sociology of Health and Illness*, 27(7), 897–919.

National Institute for health and Clinical Excellence (NICE) (2006) *The Guidelines Development Process: An Overview for Stakeholders, the Public and the NHS.* London: NICE.

Navarro, V. (1976) *Medicine Under Capitalism.* London: Croom Helm.

Navarro, V. (1986) *Crisis, Health and Medicine: A Social Critique.* London: Tavistock.

Navarro, V. (2002) A critique of social capital, *International Journal of Health Services*, 32(3), 423–432.

Nelkin, D. and Lindee, M. S. (1995) The mediated gene: Stories of gender and race. In J. Terry and J. Urla (eds) *Deviant Bodies: Critical Perspectives on Difference in Science and Popular Culture.* Bloomington, IN: Indiana University Press, 387–402.

Nettleton, S. (1991) Wisdom, diligence and teeth: Discursive practices and the creation of mothers. *Sociology of Health and Illness*, 13(1), 98–111.

Nettleton, S. (1994) Inventing mouths: Disciplinary power and dentistry. In Jones, C. and Porter, R. (eds) *Reassessing Foucault: Power, Medicine and the Body.* London and New York: Routledge, 73–90.

Nettleton, S. (1997) Governing the risky self: How to become healthy, wealthy and wise. In Petersen, A. and Bunton, R. (eds) *Foucault, Health and Medicine.* London and New York: Routledge, 207–222.

Nettleton, S. (2004) The emergence of escaped medicine? *Sociology – The Journal of the British Sociological Association*, 38(4), 661–679.

Nettleton, S., Burrows, R. and Watt, I. (2008) Regulating medical bodies? The consequences of the 'modernisation' of the NHS and the disembodiment of clinical knowledge. *Sociology of Health and Illness*, 30(3), 333–348.

Nicholson, L. (ed.) (1990) *Feminism/Postmodernism.* London: Routledge.

Nicholson, L. (1992) On the postmodern barricades: Feminism, politics and social theory. In Seidman, S. and Wagner, D. G. (eds), *Postmodernism and Social Theory*. Oxford: Basil Blackwell, 82–100.

Noddings, N. (1984) *Caring: A Feminine Approach to Ethics and Moral Education*. Berkeley: University of California Press.

Novas, C. and Rose, N. (2000) Genetic risk and the birth of the somatic individual. *Economy and Society*, 29(4), 485–513.

O'Brien, R., Hunt, K. and Hart, G. (2005) 'It's caveman stuff, but that is to a certain extent how guys still operate': Men's accounts of masculinity and help seeking. *Social Science and Medicine*, 61(3), 503–516.

O'Farrell, N. (2002) Genital ulcers, stigma, HIV and STI control in sub-Saharan Africa. *Sexually Transmitted Infections*, 78(2), 143–146.

Oakley, A (1980) *Woman Confined: Towards a Sociology of Childbirth*. Oxford: Martin Robinson.

Oakley, A. (1981) Interviewing women: A contradiction in terms. In H. Roberts (ed.), *Doing Feminist Research*. London: Routledge and Kegan Paul, 30–61.

Oakley, A. (1993) *Essays on Women, Health and Medicine*. Edinburgh: Edinburgh University Press.

Office for National Statistics (2002) *National Statistics Socio-Economic Classification (NS-SEC) for England, Scotland and Wales London: Office for National Statistics.* http://www.statistics.gov.uk/, last accessed November 2007.

Oliffe, J. (2005) Constructions of masculinity following prostatectomy-induced impotence. *Social Science and Medicine*, 60(10), 2249–2259.

Oliver, R. (1990) *The Politics of Disablement*. London: Macmillan.

Oppenheimer, M. (1973) The proletarianisation of the professional. *Sociological Review Monograph*, 20, 213–237.

Ørnstru, H. (2000) Gerog Simmel. In Andersen, H. and Bo Kaspersen, L. (eds) *Classical and Modern Social Theory*. Oxford: Blackwell, 96–108.

Osborne, T. (1997) Of health and statecraft. In Petersen, A. and Bunton, R. (eds) *Foucault, Health and Medicine*. London and New York: Routledge, 173–188.

Osler, M., Andersen, A-M. N., Due, P., Lund, R., Damsgaard, M. T. and Holstein, B. E. (2003) Socioeconomic position in early life, birth weight, childhood cognitive function, and adult mortality. A longitudinal study of Danish men born in 1953. *Journal of Epidemiology and Community Health*, 57, 681–686.

Outhwaite, W. (2005) Interpretivism and interactionism. In Harrington, A. (ed.) *Modern Social Theory: An Introduction*. Oxford: Oxford University Press, 110–131.

Paley, J. (1997) Husserl, phenomenology and nursing. *Journal of Advanced Nursing*, 26(1), 187–193.

Paley, J. (1998) Misinterpreting phenomenology: Heidegger, ontology and nursing research. *Journal of Advanced Nursing*, 27(4), 817–824.

Parker, D. and Lawton, R. (2000). Judging the use of clinical protocols by fellow professionals. *Social Science and Medicine*, 51(5), 669–677.

Parker, J. (2000) *Structuration*. Buckingham: Open University Press.

Parkin, F. (1979) *Marxism and Class Theory: A Bourgeois Critique*. London: Tavistock.

Parsons, T. (1951) *The Social System*. New York: Free Press.

Parthasarathy, S. (2005) Architectures of genetic medicine: Comparing genetic testing for breast cancer in the USA and the UK. *Social Studies of Science*, 35(1), 5–40.

Patja, A., Davidkin, I., Kurki, T., Kallio, M., Valle, M. and Peltola, H. (2000) Serious adverse events after measles-mumps-rubella vaccination during a fourteen-year prospective follow-up. *Pediatric Infectious Disease Journal*, 19(12), 1127–1134.

Pawson, R. and Tilley, S. (1997) *Realistic Evaluation*. London: Sage.

Petersen, A. (1997) Risk, governance and the new public health. In Petersen, A. and Bunton, R. (eds) *Foucault, Health and Medicine*. London and New York: Routledge, 189–206.

Petersen, A. and Bunton, R. (2002) *The New Genetics and the Public's Health*. London and New York: Routledge.

Petersen, A. and Bunton, R. (eds) (1997) *Foucault, Health and Medicine*. London and New York: Routledge.

Phillips, A. and Rausen, J. (1971) *Our Bodies Ourselves*. Penguin.

Pierret, J. (2003) The illness experience: State of knowledge and perspectives for research. *Sociology of Health and Illness*, 25(1), 2–22.

Pilnick, A. (2002) *Genetics and Society: An Introduction*. Buckingham: Open University Press.

Pinch, T. P. and Bijker, W. E. ([1987] 1990) The social construction of facts and artifacts: Or how the sociology of science and the sociology of technology might benefit each other. In Bijker, W. E., Hughes, T. P. and Pinch, T. (eds) *The Social Construction of Technological Systems: New Directions in the Sociology and History of Technology*. Cambridge, MA: MIT Press, 17–50.

Poirier, J., Delisle, M.-C., Aubert, I., Farlow, M., Lahiri, D., Hui, S. *et al.* (1995) Apolipoprotein E Allele as a Predictor of Cholinergic Deficits and Treatment Outcome in Alzheimer's Disease. *Proceedings of the National Academy of Sciences*, 92, 12260.

Pollock, A. M. (2004) *NHS plc: The Privatisation of Our Healthcare*. London: Verso.

Poloma, M. (1979) *Contemporary Sociological Theory*. London: Collier Macmillan Publishers.

Poltorak, M., Leach, M., Fairhead, J. and Cassell, J. (2005) MMR talk and vaccination choices: An ethnographic study in Brighton. *Social Science and Medicine*, 61(3), 709–719.

Popay, J., Williams, G., Thomas, C. and Gatrell, T. (1998) Theorising inequalities in health: The place of lay knowledge. *Sociology of Health and Illness*, 20(5), 619–644.

Porter, S. (1991) A participant observation study of power relations between nurses and doctors in a general hospital. *Journal of Advanced Nursing*, 16, 728–735.

Porter, S. (1992) Women in a women's job: The gendered experience of nurses. *Sociology of Health and Illness*, 14(4), 510–527.

Porter, S. (1995a) Northern nursing: The limits of idealism. *Irish Journal of Sociology*, 5, 22–42.

Porter, S. (1995b) Sociology and the nursing curriculum: A defence. *Journal of Advanced Nursing*, 21(6), 1130–1135.

Porter, S. (1996) Qualitative research. In Cormack, F. S. (ed.) *The Research Process in Nursing* (3rd edition). Oxford: Blackwell Science, 113–122.

Porter, S. (1996a) Real bodies, real needs: A critique of the application of Foucault's philosophy to nursing. *Social Sciences in Health*, 2(4), 218–227.

Porter, S. (1996b) Contra-Foucault: Soldiers, nurses and power. *Sociology*, 30(1), 59–78.

Porter, S. (1998) *Social Theory and Nursing Practice*. London: Palgrave.

Porter, S. (2001) Nightingale's realist philosophy of science. *Nursing Philosophy*, 2(1), 14–25.

Portes, A. (1998) Social capital: Its origins and applications in modern sociology. *Annual Review of Sociology*, 24(1), 1–24.

Poulton, R., Caspi, A., Milne B. J., Thomson, M. W., Taylor, A., Sears, M. R. and Moffitt, T. E. (2002) Association between children's experience of socioeconomic disadvantage and adult health: A life-course study. *Lancet*, 360(9346), 1640–1645.

Press, N., Reynolds, S., Pinsky, L., Murthy, V., Leo, M. and Burke, W. (2005) 'That's like chopping off a finger because you're afraid it might get broken': Disease and illness in women's views of prophylactic mastectomy. *Social Science and Medicine*, 61(5), 1106–1117.

Putnam, R. (1993) *Making Democracy Work: Civic Traditions in Modern Italy*. New Jersey: Princeton University Press.

Putnam, R. (1995) Bowling alone: America's declining social capital. *Journal of Democracy*, 6(1), 65–78.

Putnam, R. (2000) *Bowling Alone: The Collapse and Revival of American Community*. New York: Simon & Schuster.

Radley, A. (1994) *Making Sense of Illness. The Social Psychology of Health and Disease*. Sage: London.

Rappert, B. and Brown, N. (2000) Putting the future in its place: Comparing innovation moments in genetic diagnostics and telemedicine. *New Genetics and Society*, 19(1), 49–74.

Rich, A. (1977) *Of Woman Born*. London: Virago.

Ridgeway, C. L. and Smith-Lovin, L. (1999) The gender system and interaction. *Annual Review of Sociology*, 25, 191–216.

Ritzer, G. and Goodman, D. J. (2003) *Sociological Theory* (6th edition). Boston: McGraw Hill.

Robertson, S. (2006a) 'Not living life in too much of an excess': Lay men understanding health and well-being. *Health*, 10(2), 175–189.

Robertson, S. (2006b) 'I've been like a coiled spring this last week': Embodied masculinity and health. *Sociology of Health and Illness*, 28(4), 433–456.

Rose, N. ([1989] 1999) *Governing the Soul: The Shaping of the Private Self* (2nd edition). London and New York: Free Association Books.

Rose, S. (1995) The rise of neurogenetic determinism. *Nature*, 373, 380–382.

Rosenfeld, D. and Faircloth, C. A. (2006) *Medicalized Masculinities*. Philadelphia: Temple University Press.

Rosenhan, D. L. (1973) On being sane in insane places. *Science*, 179, 250–258.

Rossi, A. (1977) A biosocial perspective on parenting. *Daedalus*, 106, 9–31.

Rossi, A. (1983) Gender and parenthood. *American Sociological Review*, 49(1), 1–19.

Roter, D. (2000) The enduring and evolving nature of the patient-physician relationship. *Patient Education and Counselling*, 39, 5–15.

Sætnan, A. R. (2000) Women's involvement with reproductive medicine: Introducing shared concepts. In Sætnan, A. R., Oudshoorn, N. and Kirejczyk, M. (eds) *Bodies of Technology: Women's Involvement with Reproductive Medicine*. Columbus: Ohio State University Press, 1–30.

Sahlins, M. (1993) *Waiting for Foucault*. Cambridge: Prickly Pear Press.

Sandstrom, K. L., Martin, D. D. and Alan Fine, G. (2001) Symbolic interactionism at the end of the century. In Ritzer, G. and Smart, B. (eds) *Handbook of Social Theory*. London: Sage, 217–231.

Sarantakos, S. (1998) *Social Research* (2nd edition). London: Macmillan.

Scambler, G. (1989) *Epilepsy*. London: Tavistock.

Scambler, G. (2001a) Critical realism, sociology and health inequalities: Social class as a generative mechanism and its media of enactment. *Journal of Critical Realism*, 4(1), 35–42.

Scambler, G. (2001b) Introduction: Unfolding themes of an incomplete project. In Scambler, G. (ed.) *Habermas, Critical Theory and Health*. London: Routledge, 1–24.

Scambler, G. (2002) *Health and Social Change: A Critical Theory*. Buckingham: Open University Press.

Scambler, G. (2004) Re-framing stigma: Felt and enacted stigma and challenges to the sociology of chronic and disabling conditions. *Social Theory and Health*, 2, 29–46.

Scambler, G. and Hopkins, A. (1986) Being epileptic: Coming to terms with stigma. *Sociology of Health and Illness*, 8(1), 26–43.

Scambler, G., Scambler, A. and Craig, D. (1981) Kinship and friendship networks and women's demand for primary care. *Journal of the Royal College of General Practitioners*, 31(233), 746–750.

Scheff, T. J. (1974) The labelling theory of mental illness. *American Sociological Review*, 39(June), 444–452.

Schiebinger, L. (1989) *The Mind Has No Sex?: Women in the Origins of Modern Science*. Cambridge, MA: Harvard University Press.

Schiebinger, L. (2003a) Skelettestreit. *Isis*, 94(2), 274–299.

Schiebinger, L. (2003b) Women's health and clinical trials. *The Journal of Clinical Investigation*, 112(7), 973–977.

Schutz, A. ([1967] 2002) The phenomenology of the social world. In Calhoun, C., Gerteis, J., Moody, J., Pfaff, S. and Virk, I. (eds) *Contemporary Sociological Theory*. Oxford: Blackwell, 32–41.

Scott, J. (2006) *Social Theory: Central issues in Sociology*. London. Thousand Oaks, New Delhi: Sage.

Shaw, M., Dorling, D. and Mitchell, R. (2002) *Health, Place and Society*. London: Prentice Hall.

Shaw, M., Dorling, D., Gordon, D. and Davey-Smith, G. (1999) *The Widening Gap: Health Inequalities and Policy in Britain*. Bristol: The Policy Press.

Sherwin, S. (1992) *No Longer Patient: Feminist Ethics and Health*. Philadelphia: Temple University Press.

Simmel, G. ([1908] 1959) The problem of sociology. In K. Wolff (ed.) *Essays in Sociology, Philosophy and Aesthetics*. New York: Harper Torchbooks, 310–336.

Sinclair, S. (1997) *Making Doctors*. Oxford: Berg.

Sismondo, S. (2004) *An Introduction to Science and Technology Studies*. Oxford: Blackwell.

Smith, B. and Sparkes, A. C. (2005) Men, sport, spinal cord injury, and narratives of hope. *Social Science and Medicine*, 61, 1095–1105.

Smith, D. (1988) *The Everyday World as Problematic: A Feminist Sociology*. Toronto: University of Toronto Press.

Snedden, R. (2000) The Challenge of pharmacogenetics and pharmacogenomics. *New Genetics and Society*, 19(2), 145–164.

Spallone, P. (1989) *Beyond Conception: The New Politics of Reproduction*. London: Macmillan.

Stafford, M., Cummins, S., Macintyre, S., Ellaway, A. and Marmot, M. (2005) Gender differences in the associations between health and neighbourhood environment. *Social Science and Medicine*, 60(6), 1168–1192.

Stein, L. (1967) The doctor-nurse game. *Archives of General Psychiatry*, 16, 699–703.

Stein, L., Watts, D. and Howell, T. (1990) The doctor-nurse game revisited. *Nursing Outlook*, 36, 264–268.

Steingart, R. M., Packer, M., Mamm, P., Coglianese, M. E., Gersh, B., Geltman, E. M., Sollano, J., Katz, S., Moye, L., Basta, L. L. *et al.* (1991) Sex differences in the management of coronary artery disease: Survival and ventricular enlargement investigators. *The New England Journal of Medicine*, 325(4), 226–230.

Stewart, M., Brown, J. B., Weston, W., Mc Whinney, I. R., McWilliam, C. I. and Freeman, T. R. (2003) *Patient Centred Medicine: Transforming the Clinical Method* (2nd edition). Oxford: Radcliff Medical Press.

Stoeckle, J. D. (1987) Working on the factory floor. *Annals of Internal Medicine*, 107(2), 250–251.

Strauss, A. L. (1978) *Negotiations: Varieties Contexts, Processes and Social Order*. London: Jossey-Bass.

Strauss, A. L. and Corbin, J. (1990) *Basics of Qualitative Research: Grounded Theory Procedures and Techniques*. London: Sage.

Strauss, A. L., Ehrlick, D., Bucher, R. and Sabshin, M. ([1963] 1998) The hospital and its negotiated order. In Mackay, L., Soothill, K. and Melia, K. (eds) *Classic Texts in Healthcare*. Oxford: Butterworth Heinemann, 248–250.

Svensson, R. (1996) The interplay between doctors and nurses – a negotiated order perspective. *Sociology of Health and Illness*, 18(93), 379–398.

Swain, J., Finkelstein, V., French, S. and Oliver, M. (eds) (1993) *Disabling Barriers – Enabling Environments*. London: Sage.

Szreter, S. and Woolcock, M. (2004) Health by association? Social capital, social theory, and the political economy of public health. *International Journal of Epidemiology*, 33(4), 650–667.

Szymczak, J. E. and Conrad, P. (2006) Medicalizing the aging male body: Andropause and baldness. In Rosenfield, D. and Faircoth, C. A. (eds) *Medicalized Masculinities*. Philadelphia: Temple University Press, 89–111.

Takahashi, M. and Kai, I. (2005) Sexuality after breast cancer treatment: Changes and coping strategies among Japanese survivors. *Social Science and Medicine*, 61(6), 1278–1290.

Taylor, S. D. (2004) Predictive genetic test decisions for Huntington's disease: Context, appraisal and new moral imperatives. *Social Science and Medicine*, 58(1), 137–149.

Taylor-Gooby, P. and Zinn, J. (eds) (2006) *Risk in Social Science*. Oxford: Oxford University Press.

Tew, M. (1998) *Safer Childbirth? A Critical History of Maternity Care* (2nd edition). New York: Free Association Books.

The Stationary Office (1998) *Independent Inquiry into Inequalities in Health (Acheson Report)*. London: The Stationary Office.

Thompson, D. (2001) *Radical Feminism Today*. Sage: London.

Thompson, L. (2008) The role of nursing in governmentality, biopower and population health: Family health nursing. *Health and Place*, 14(1), 76–84.

Townsend, P., Davidson, N. and Whitehead, M. (1992) *Inequalities and Health: The Black Report and the Health Divide*. Harmondsworth: Penguin.

Tunis, S. R., Hayward, R. S. A., Wilson, M. C., Rubin, H. R., Bass, E. B., Johnston, M. and Steinberg, E. P. (1994) Internists' attitudes about clinical practice guidelines. *Annals of Internal Medicine*, 120, 956–963.

Turner, B. (2003) Social capital, inequality and health. *Social Theory and Health*, 1(1), 4–20.

Turner, B. S. (1992) *Regulating Bodies: Essays in Medical Sociology*. London and New York: Routledge.

Turney, J. and Turner, J. (2000) Predictive medicine, genetics and schizophrenia. *New Genetics and Society*, 19(1), 5–22.

Turris, S. A. (2005) Unpacking the concept of patient satisfaction: A feminist analysis. *Journal of Advanced Nursing*, 50(3), 293–298.

Ungerson, C. (1987) *Policy Is Personal: Sex Gender and Informal Care*. London: Tavistock.

van Lente, H. (1993) *Promising technology: The Dynamics of Expectations in Technological Development*. Enschede: Department of Philosophy of Science and Technology University of Twente.

Veenstra, G. (2000) Social capital, SES and health: An individual level analysis. *Social Science and Medicine*, 50(5), 619–629.

Wakefield, A. J., Murch, S. H., Anthony, A., Linnell, J., Casson, D. M., Malik, M., Berelowitz, M., Dillion, A. P., Thompson, M. A., Harvey, P., Valentine, A., Davies, S. E. and Walker-Smith, J. A. (1998) Ileal-lymphoid-nodular hyperplasis, non-specific colitis, and pervasive developmental disorder in children. *Lancet*, 351, 637–641.

Walby, S. and Greenwell, J. (1994) *Medicine and Nursing: Professions in a Changing Health Service*. London: Sage.

Weber, M. ([1922] 1978) *Economy and Society: An Outline of Interpretative Sociology*. New York, Bedminster Press.

Weber, M. (1970) Class, status and party. In Gerth, H. and Mills, C. (eds) *From Max Weber: Essays in Sociology*. London: Routledge and Kegan Paul, 180–195.

Weber, M. ([1947] 2002) Basic sociological terms. In Calhoun, C., Gerteis, J., Moody, J., Pfaff, S., Schmidt, K. and Virk, I. (eds) *Classical Sociological Theory*. Oxford: Blackwell, 178–187.

Weber, M. (1978 [1922]) *Economy and Society: Volumes 1 and 2*. G. Roth and C. Wittich (eds). Berkeley and Los Angeles: University of California Press.

Webster, A. (1991) *Science, Technology and Society*. London: Macmillan.

Werner, A. and Malterud, K. (2003) It is hard work behaving as a credible patient: Encounters between women with chronic pain and their doctors. *Social Science and Medicine*, 57(8), 1409–1419.

Werner, A., Widding Isaksen, L. and Malterud, K. (2004) 'I am not the kind of women who complains of everything': Illness stories on self and shame in women with chronic pain. *Social Science and Medicine*, 59(5), 1035–1045.

Wharton, A. S. (2005) *The Sociology of Gender: An Introduction to Theory and Research*. Oxford: Blackwell Publishing.

Wickrama, K. A. S., Lorenz, F. O., Conger, R. D., Elder, G. H., Abraham, W. T. and Fang, S. (2006) Changes in family financial circumstances and the physical health of married and recently divorced mothers. *Social Science and Medicine*, 63(1), 123–136.

Wicks, D. (1998) *Nurses and Doctors at Work: Rethinking Professional Boundaries*. Buckingham: Open University Press.

Widerberg, K. (2000) Gender and society. In Andersen, H. and Bo Kaspersen, L. (eds) *Classical and Modern Social Theory*. Oxford: Blackwell, 467–487.

Wilkinson R. (1996) *Unhealthy Societies: The Afflictions of Inequality*. London: Routledge.

Wilkinson, R. (1999) The culture of inequality. In Kawachi, B., Kennedy, B. and Eilkinson, R. (eds) *Income Inequality and Health: The Society and Population Reader, Vol. 1*. New York: New Press.

Wilkinson, R. G. and Pickett, K. E. (2006) Income Inequality and population health: A review and explanation of the evidence. *Social Science and Medicine*, 62(7), 1768–1784.

Williams, C., Sandall, J., Lewando-Hundt, G., Heyman, B., Spencer, K. and Grellier, R. (2005) Women as moral pioneers? Experiences of first trimester antenatal screening. *Social Science and Medicine*, 61(9), 1983–1992.

Williams, G. (1984) The genesis of chronic illness: Narrative reconstruction. *Sociology of Health and Illness*, 6, 175–200.

Williams, S. (1999) Is anybody there? Critical realism, chronic illness and the disability debate. *Sociology of Health and Illness*, 21(6), 797–819.

Williams, S. and Bendelow, G. (1998) *The Lived Body: Sociological Themes, Embodied Issues*. London: Routledge.

Williams-Jones, B. and Graham, J. (2003) Actor-network theory: A tool to support ethical analysis of commercial genetic testing. *New Genetics and Society*, 22(3), 272–296.

Winch, S., Creedy, D. and Chaboyer, W. (2002) Governing nursing conduct: The rise of evidence-based practice. *Nursing Inquiry*, 9(3), 156–161.

Wollstonecraft, M. (1792) *Vindication of the Rights of Women*. Penguin Classics published in 1992.

Yuill, C. (2005) Marx: Capitalism, alienation and health. *Social Theory and Health*, 3, 126–143.

Zibbel, J. E. (2004) Can the lunatics actually take over the asylum? Reconfiguring subjectivity and neo-liberal governance in contemporary British drug treatment policy. *International Journal of Drug Policy*, 15(1), 56–65.

Ziersch, A. M. (2005) Health implications of access to social capital: Findings from an Australian Study. *Social Science and Medicine*, 61(10), 2119–2131.

Zola, I. K. (1972) Medicine as an institution of social control. *Sociological Review*, 20, 487–504.

Index

In this index, tables are indicated in **bold**. Notes are indicated by n. Published works are entered in *italics*.